A Handbook of Yoga-Nidrā

A Handbook of Yoga-Nidrā

Kamakhya Kumar

With a foreword by
Pranav Pandya

DK PRINTWORLD
Publishers of Indian Traditions

Cataloging in Publication Data — DK
[Courtesy: D.K. Agencies (P) Ltd. <docinfo@dkagencies.com>]

Kāmākhyā Kumāra, 1975- author.
A handbook of yoga-nidrā/ Kamakhya Kumar; with a foreword by Pranav Pandya.
p. cm.
Includes bibliographical references (p.) and index.
ISBN 9788124606858

1. Yoga. 2. Meditation. 3. Spiritual life – Hinduism. 4. Yoga – Therapeutic use. 5. Relaxation. I. Title.

DDC 181.45 23

First published in India, 2013
Second Impression in 2019
ISBN 13: 978-81-246-0685-8 (HB) ISBN 10: 81-246-0685-4
ISBN 13: 978-81-246-0686-5 (PB) ISBN 10: 81-246-0686-2

Printed and published by:
D.K. Printworld (P) Ltd.
Regd. office : Vedaśrī, F-395, Sudarshan Park
(Metro Station: ESI Hospital) New Delhi - 110 015
Phones : (011) 2545 3975, 2546 6019
e-mail : indology@dkprintworld.com
Web : www.dkprintworld.com

Dedicated to
My Mother

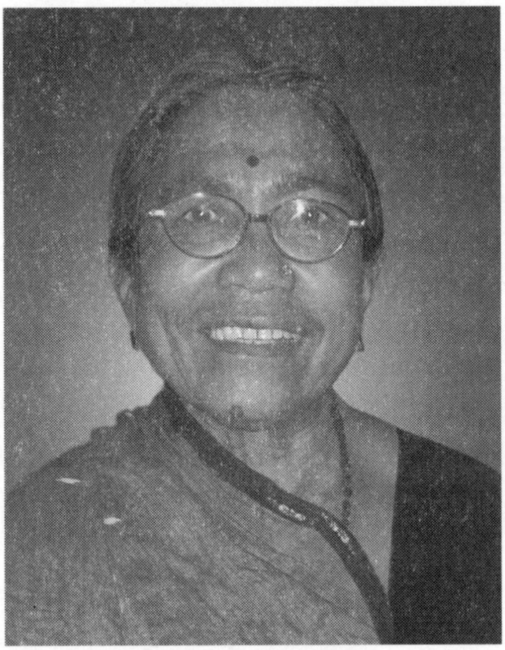

Late Srimati Indu Devi
(1939–2010)

Foreword

YOGA has become a buzzword now allover. The whole world is now accepting *yoga*. The Indian scientists of the Vedic Age had devised the *sādhanā* of *yoga-nidrā* and *samādhi*, which served the purpose of self-analysis and self-development simultaneously. These *sādhanā* practices are risk-less and effective as they are naturally adaptive as per the physical and mental health, intrinsic nature and spiritual level of practitioners.

Yoga-nidrā is one of the most powerful and time-tested spiritual techniques to go beyond the body consciousness and experience the subconscious and later on the superconscious states of the self. In this stage, the individual consciousness enters the subtlest, the innermost and the divine core of life — the sheath of ultimate bliss. Realization of the soul and the absolute linkage with the cosmic consciousness can be attained in this state. Divine messages are received in such condition that inspires sublime transmutation of the individual self.

A Handbook of Yoga-Nidrā presents the invaluable pearls of ancient knowledge and the deeper aspect of creative conjugation of mind with the inner impulses of the soul. It introduces the history, philosophy and all psycho-physiological aspects of *yoga-nidrā* explaining how it works in both yogic and scientific terms. It includes several scientific studies particularly the multidirectional approaches of this unique relaxation technique, on the basis of modern medical as well as psychological tools.

The progress of this *sādhanā*, as described in this book, results not only in better physiological and psychological condition of the body and mind, it also reflects into gradual arousal of hidden potentials of spiritual transmutation. It is hoped that the book would be interesting and informative to all those who are interested in yogic knowledge. It will be of great use to graduates, postgraduates and research students, and teachers of the *yoga* and allied system of therapy.

I wish Kamakhya Kumar, great success, who has made a wonderful effort to bring this vast knowledge of *yoga-nidrā* into a lucid form through this book.

14 January 2013 **Pranav Pandya**

Preface

THE entire Vedic literature, and the sages and savants of the Śāstric scriptures have given paramount importance to *yoga* and have discussed in detail the methods of the yogic practices. There is no scripture, which does not sing paeans of the pre-eminent benefits and supramental effects of this time-tested method that encompasses the personal, global and the cosmic realms of existence.

It is said that even if one performs *dhyāna* (meditation) with fervent faith without going through all the prescribed ascetic disciplines of higher-level *sādhanā*s, he attains some of the benefits of *yoga sādhanā*. From the perspective of the studies conducted worldwide, it can be inferred that yogic practices influence the human physiology. Not only the physiological aspect, the psychological and the spiritual cores of this practice are also so sound that it appears to be founded on profound scientific basis.

In day-to-day life, individuals fail to express their emotions freely and openly. As a result, the emotions are repressed and manifest in the form of emotional tension. Due to excessive activity on the mental plane, the mind always remains in a state of arousal, which results in mental tension. Throughout life the mind is fed with negative data. The shadows of cultural anarchy, tribulation, fright and disharmony seen in the social fronts also make collective reflections of the inner disharmony, fear, desperation, insecurity, despair, jealousy, discontentment, suppressed desires, etc. at the individual levels.

At the root of all these devilish drives lie the ghostly complexities of ignorant, perverted and shattered minds. The accelerating rates of psychosomatic diseases and personality disorders are causes of serious concern and have posed an unprecedented challenge to human intellect and consciousness.

Yoga-nidrā helps to restore mental, emotional and physical health by way of relaxation, and makes the mind more conducive to *pratyāhāra* (withdrawing senses from their objects), *dhāraṇā* (concentration) and meditation. This practice helps to harmonize the two hemispheres of the brain, and both the sympathetic and parasympathetic aspects of autonomous nervous system — the impressions in the subconscious are brought to surface, experienced and removed. Thus, the fixation of awareness to the body is replaced with an awareness of the subtler aspects of *prāṇa* and spiritual dimensions.

Through the practice of *yoga-nidrā*, the practitioners slowly moves towards the deeper realms of the mind where they confront their deep-rooted emotional tensions. When the practitioner recognizes these emotional tensions with full awareness and a witnessing attitude, repressed emotions are released, and the practitioner becomes calm and tranquil.

In the practice of *yoga-nidrā*, especially in rotation of consciousness and breath awareness, the mind is relaxed, thereby releasing the mental tensions. In this way, through the regular and sincere practice of *yoga-nidrā*, tensions at the physical, emotional and mental levels can be minimized.

Good health is one of the greatest resources for vitality, creativity and wealth, while poor health in contrast significantly drains them. The good old days have gone when health was synonymous with the absence of disease, and all that was needed to assign us with a "healthy" or "unhealthy" label was a visit to the doctor's office. Many killer diseases of the past such as measles and tuberculosis, caused by pathogens or germs, flourished in the poor environmental conditions of the past.

The psychological crisis of this age is perhaps the severest of the crises human race has ever faced. Considering at the severity of the psychological complications found in majority of people today, it looks difficult to reverse the subtle but the fast decline of human health (and hence the existence of human civilization) towards pathetic extinction.

Normally, an average person can tolerate a certain amount of psychic trauma without much disturbance. However, if it exceeds the limit of his endurance various psychological changes take place. Normally, such a phase remains in the body for a short while. If it becomes recurrent in the form of a repeated psychic trauma, then one may observe some visible and demonstrable changes in the behaviour and personality of the person. Anxiety, stress, regression, guilt, arousal and fatigue are the manifestations of the behavioural and personality disorders.

Whenever a psychological or physiological stress occurs, the entire psychosomatic apparatus of our body tries to adapt itself in order to face external environmental challenges more effectively and successfully. Entire body chemistry changes within seconds. As the result of sympathetic arousal, imbalance and disharmony in the functioning of internal organs occur. This demanding situation of the body increases the respiration rate as well as the pulse rate. The stressed condition of the body results in vaso-spasm, the muscles become stiff as the blood supply in the arteries becomes difficult, which results into high blood pressure. In this situation there occurs increased activity of the cerebral cortex, especially of the psychic centre. This can be observed by the electroencephalogram (EEG) changes and biochemical changes of the body.

The mechanisms of action of the psychic, somatic and visceral centres of our brain are closely interconnected by efficient anatomical and physiological links. However, the psychic centres are more closely associated with somatic centres than the autonomically-controlled visceral centres. Thus psychological disorders such as lack of memory and lack of well-being of the person can be observed.

The international problem today is not hunger, poverty, drugs or fear of war, it is only mental imbalances — and their manifestations in the form of psychosomatic diseases. These inner tensions of the individual can only be dealt with inner peace. The yogic texts all unequivocally state that peace can only be found within never without, therefore to create a more peaceful world, we must first learn how to relax and harmonize our own body and mind.

Ancient Indian saints as well as contemporary *yogī*s have established a wonderful relaxation technique, called *yoga-nidrā*. There are several techniques to relax the body and mind, but *yoga-nidrā* is probably the best-known technique to induce complete physical, mental and emotional relaxation. It is a method of peeling off the subliminal sheath of conscious (external) mind that covers the inner core of the unconscious (inner) mind. In this state, the individual consciousness is able to receive the cosmic signals of the superconsciousness. *Yoga-nidrā* aims at the removal of the *pratyaya* (mental fluctuations) from the conscious or external plane, the subconscious or subtle plane and the unconscious or causal plane. *Yoga-nidrā* is a state between sleep and *samādhi*. It is a half sleep and half waking state. This simple and useful practice of the art of sleeping which the *yogī*s know may be called psychic sleep.

Since this is the age of scientific investigation, nothing can be believed without proof. This is the time to go deep into the search of its physiological and psychological impact on our body and mind, and on the basis of that a more applicable form of *yoga-nidrā* can be given to the society. At its simplest level, it may be understood and practised as a way of total physical and mental relaxation. The advanced benefits can be reached with regular practice.

Although *yoga-nidrā* is of great help to insomniacs because it stimulates sleep, it must be understood that *yoga-nidrā* itself is not sleep. At best, it can be described as "sleep of awareness". In conventional sleep, we lose control of our senses. But if someone seeks the greatest benefits, one must transcend this feeling so that one can stimulate the mind in the desired manner and be under control.

Various studies have been done in different parts of the world for observing the effect of *yoga-nidrā*. *Yoga-nidrā* has been experienced as "the" most powerful relaxation technique known to man. Yet, in *yoga*, it is used much more than that. The power of this technique is such that it is regularly used as a therapeutic technique to overcome pain, neurosis and even disability in certain cases.

Kamakhya Kumar

Contents

1

History of Yoga-Nidrā

THE beginning of the *yoga* tradition is undoubtedly shrouded in the mystery of antiquity, but it is universally recognized that Indian *yoga* constitutes one of the oldest and most important scientific spiritual legacies of humanity and has been preached as well as practised uninterruptedly since the dawn of human history.

Some scholars are of the opinion that the divine tradition of *yoga* began with the very resonance of Vedic *ṛcā* (*mantras*) in the caves of Devātmā Himalayas. With the very first ray of civilization the divine light of *yoga* spread in human life. The essence of the divine knowledge of the ancient seers lies in this very *yoga*.

Even the *Ṛgveda,* which is the oldest book in the world, speaks of *mantras* regarding yogic practices. *Mantras* like 10.177.1 of the *Ṛgveda* and 10.2.30-32, 10.8.83 of the *Atharvaveda* bear testimony to this fact. It covers almost every step of *yoga* in different contexts.

We have the description of different processes of *yoga* in *Aitareya Āraṇyaka* 2.17, 3.1, 3.4, 3.6; *Taittirīya Āraṇyaka* 2.2, 2.7, 2.9; *Śatapatha Brāhmaṇa* 1.4.4.7, 14.3.2.3; and *Taittirīya Brāhmaṇa* 3.10.18.6, 1.2.6. On the other, we find the growth of certain yogic tenets in the Brāhmaṇas like *Kauṣītaki, Jaiminīya* and *Gopatha.* In these we get elaborate description of *prāṇa-vidyā* and advanced ideas regarding *prāṇa-vidyā*. *Praṇava* is another technical name for *oṁ.*

There are several Upaniṣads like *Kena, Kaṭha, Kauṣītaki, Praśna, Muṇḍaka, Māṇḍūkya, Taittirīya, Aitareya, Chāndogya, Bṛhadāraṇyaka* and *Śvetāśvatara* which reflect *yoga* in one form or the other. *Yoga-nidrā* comes in for the first time in *Māṇḍūkyopaniṣad.*

Anyone who reads them in the original Sanskrit is caught up and carried away by the elevation, profundity and compelling fascination of the pregnant, often poetic utterances through which they unravel the mysterious and sacred relations of the human soul with the ultimate reality. Arthur Schopenhauer was among the leading German philosophers of the last century who got acquainted with some early Upaniṣads through a Latin rendering from a personal translation. He was so impressed and moved by what he read in them that he wrote the following inspiring and oft-quoted words — an English translation of his German outpouring:

> Upaniṣads like *Chāndogya* and *Bṛhadāraṇyaka* which reflect the basis of *kriyā-yoga, prāṇa* and *nāḍīs* are important topics discussed here. In *Kaṭhopaniṣad* the word *yoga* has been used in its technical sense, whereas in Upaniṣads like *Īśa, Kena* and *Kaṭha* we have the information on the firm basis of *yoga.*[1]

In fact, *Śvetāśvatara Upaniṣad* is regarded as the most authentic book on *yoga-vidyā* as it describes the essence of yogic practices and their physiological effects.

We have the description of *yoga* even in great Indian epics like the *Rāmāyaṇa* and the *Mahābhārata.* These epics are the rich sources of information about various kinds of yogic practices, but the term *yoga-nidrā* doesn't come as it is.

We have the description of the importance of *yoga* in Śrutis (the essence of Vedas known through aural transmission), Smṛtis and Purāṇas, but we couldn't find the term *yoga-nidrā* in this period.

As well understood and appreciated by serious students of *yoga*, the *Yoga-Sūtras* consist of just 196 short statements or aphorism (*sūtras*), divided into four sections entitled *samādhi* (unitive experience), *sādhanā* (spiritual practice), *vibhūti* (para-

---

[1] *The Philosophy of the Upanishads,* Suresh Chandra Chakravarti.

normal attainments) and *kaivalya* (self-realization). According to tradition, this work was composed by Patañjali, whose date is uncertain, but is believed to have lived around 300 BCE.

The period of Smṛti literature starts from the time of Patañjali, some Smṛtis had been composed before 500 BCE and they were written till about CE 1000. During this long period of Smṛti literature, we find the changes in the travelling of ideas, beliefs, worships and customs. The Smṛtis tried to combine *yoga* with the daily rituals. Thus we find *prāṇāyāma* and certain purificatory techniques occupying an important place in every ritual.

Thus Patañjali's *Yoga-Sūtras* is the oldest, systematic treatise on *yoga* available to us. It is based on the previous and contemporary traditions of *yoga*. Several commentaries have been written on the *Yoga-Sūtras* of Patañjali which throw light on the development of different yogic concepts and techniques of that period. Almost every aspect of yoga has been well defined in Patañjali's *Yoga-Sūtras*, even *nidrā* has been well defined as a *vṛtti*, but *yoga-nidrā* couldn't appear in this text.

Yoga-nidrā was first discussed in *Durgā Saptaśatī*, one of the parts of the great, *Mārkaṇḍeya Purāṇa*. According to the visualizations of Maharṣi Mārkaṇḍeya "at the end of *kalpa* when the entire universe was in a deep relaxation Lord Viṣṇu was laying on the bed of a serpent in the state of *yoga-nidrā*". He states in his Purāṇa that Lordess Yoga-Nidrā lives in the eyes of Lord Viṣṇu. When Lord Brahmā observed Him in the state of *yoga-nidrā*, to make him awake, He (Brahmā) started praying to the Lordess Yoga-Nidrā.

Later on *Haṭha-Yoga Pradīpikā* (4.49) took this term *yoga-nidrā* as a means of *samādhi*. Even then the practical aspect of *yoga-nidrā* didn't come into focus.

Great Yogī Ādya Śaṅkarācārya explained *yoga-nidrā* for the first time in a very specific manner in his text *Yoga Tārāvalī* (verses 25-26). This one was the real *yoga-nidrā* with its all quintessentials. We have mentioned them all in the next chapter.

Later on in 1975 onwards Swami Satyananda Saraswati, Swami Rama and Pandit Sri Ram Sharma Acharya developed their own techniques and spread the knowledge of *yoga-nidrā* in an applicable form. This was the beginning of *yoga-nidrā* for a society. Afterwards came the implementation and application of this marvellous technique for the betterment of human life.

A number of researches have been done in this area and many books and articles have been published to observe and practise the physiological, psychological and therapeutic effects of *yoga-nidrā* in the last few decades. In the year 2006, one of the PhD theses "Psycho-physiological Changes as Related to Yoga-Nidrā" was one of the notable works in the field of yogic science, as it was the result of six months' observation on several specific aspects of this practice. The findings are also discussed in detail in the following chapters.

2

Yoga-Nidrā in Scriptures

SCRIPTURE or Purāṇas are a group of important Indian texts, notably consisting of narratives of the history of the Universe from creation to destruction, genealogies of the kings, heroes, sages and demi-gods, and descriptions of Indian cosmology, philosophy and geography. Purāṇas usually give prominence to a particular deity and most of them use abundant religious and philosophical concepts. They are usually written in the form of stories related to one person or another.

The date of the production of the written texts does not give the date of origin of the Purāṇas, for on one hand they unquestionably existed, in some oral form a millennium before, while on the other hand they have been incrementally modified well into medieval times and perhaps down to the present day.

An early reference is found in the *Chāndogya Upaniṣad* 7.1.2 (*c.* 500 BCE). The *Bṛhadāraṇyaka Upaniṣad* refers to Purāṇa as the "fifth Veda": *itihāsapurāṇam pañcamam vedānām*, reflecting the early religious importance of these ideas, presumably then in purely oral form. The term also appears in the *Atharvaveda* 11.7.24· According to *Matysa Purāṇa*, they are said to narrate five subjects, called *pañcalakṣaṇa* (five distinguishing marks):

1. *Sarga*: The creation of the universe.
2. *Pratisarga*: Secondary creations, mostly recreations after dissolution.
3. *Vaṁśa*: Genealogy of gods and sages.
4. *Manvantara*: The creation of the human race and the first human beings. The epoch of the Manu's rule, 71 celestial *yuga*s or 308,448,000 years.
5. *Vaṁśānucaritam*: Dynastic histories.

The Purāṇas also lay emphasis on keeping a record of genealogies. The *Vāyu Purāṇa* says: "In ancient times the *sūta*'s duty was to preserve the genealogies of gods, *ṛṣis* and glorious kings, and the traditions of great men." The Purāṇic genealogies indicate that Manu Vaivasvata lived ninety-five generations before the Mahābhārata War.

Although these texts are related to each other, and material in one is found in another, they nevertheless each present a view of ordering of the world from a particular perspective. They must not be seen as random collections of old tales, but as highly selective and crafted expositions and presentations of world-views and soteriologies, compiled by particular groups of brāhmaṇas to propagate a particular vision, whether it be focused on Viṣṇu, Śiva, or Devī, or, indeed, any number of deities.

The Purāṇas are available in vernacular translations and are disseminated by brāhmaṇa scholars, who read from them and tell their stories, usually in *kathā* sessions (in which a travelling brāhmaṇa settles for a few weeks in a temple and narrates parts of a Purāṇa, usually with a *bhakti* perspective).

The *Mārkaṇḍeya Purāṇa,* one of the major eighteen Purāṇas, a Hindu religious text, is in the style of a dialogue between the sages Jaiminī and Mārkaṇḍeya. It has no sectarian content, that is, it is neutral to Viṣṇu and Śiva, and other aspects of the deities. It begins with the four questions put forth by Jaiminī to Mārkaṇḍeya. The text is consisted of 134 chapters. The chapters 50-97 contain the accounts of the fourteen *manvantara*s (the periods of the Manus) of which thirteen chapters (chapters 78-90) are together known as *Devī Māhātmya.*

The *Devī Māhātmya* (Sanskrit: *Devimāhātmyam* or "Glory of the Goddess") is a Hindu text describing the victory of the Goddess Durgā over the demon Mahiṣāsura. As part of the *Mārkaṇḍeya Purāṇa,* it is one of the Purāṇas or secondary Hindu scriptures, and was composed in Sanskrit around *c.* CE 400-500, with the authorship attributed to the sage Mārkaṇḍeya.

Devimāhātmyam is also known as the *Durgā Saptaśatī* or simply *Saptaśatī, Caṇḍī* or *Caṇḍī Pāṭha* — where *pāṭha* (reading) refers to the act of ritual reading. The text contains 700 (*saptaśata* — "seven hundred") verses, arranged into thirteen chapters. By far the most important text of Śāktism, the text has a central place in Śākta ritual.

Devimāhātmyam is seen as an attempt to unify the Vedic male pantheon with the pre-existing Mother Goddess cult possibly dating to the ninth millennium BCE, and an attempt to define divinity as a *female principle*. The text synthesizes a number of pre-existing Mother Goddess myths of Aryan and non-Aryan origins, skilfully integrated into a single narrative. The position of the Goddess as Śakti, power itself, beyond the patriarchal position as *consort* of an eclipsing male deity, is an important transition in Hindu mythology. Also, there are links to aspects of Sāṁkhya philosophy in the narrative.

For ritual reading purposes a number of subsidiary texts are appended before and after. A ritual reading of this text is part of the Navarātri celebrations in honour of the goddess. In eastern India, the ritual reading (*Caṇḍī Pāṭha*) is common at several functions, particularly in death rites.

According to Maharṣi Mārkaṇḍeya, *yoga-nidrā* is the state of deep relaxation as Lord Viṣṇu Himself used this marvellous technique:

उत्पन्नेति तदा लोके सा नित्याप्यभिधीयते।
योगनिद्रां यदा विष्णुर्जगत्येकार्णवीकृते।।६६।।

utpanneti tadā loke sā nityāpyabhidhīyate ।
yoga-nidrāṁ yadā viṣṇurjagatyekārṇavīkṛte ॥

— *Durgāsaptaśati* 1.66

Maharṣi Mārkaṇḍeya according to his visualizations states in his text the *Mārkaṇḍeya Purāṇa* that at the end of *kalpa* when the entire universe was in a state of deep relaxation, Lord Viṣṇu was lying on the bed of a serpent in the state of *yogā-nidrā*.

दृष्ट्वा. तावसुरौ चोग्रौ प्रसुप्तं च जनार्दनम्।
तुष्टाव योगनिद्रां तामेकाग्रहृदयस्थितः।।६९।।

draṣṭvā tāvasurau cograu prasuptaṁ ca janārdanam ।
tuṣṭāva yoga-nidrāṁ tāmekāgrahṛdyasthitaḥ ॥

— *Durgāsaptśati* 1.69

When Lord Brahmā observed Him in the state of *yoga-nidrā,* to make him awake, He started praying to the Lordess Yoga-Nidrā which lives in the eye of Lord Viṣṇu.

In ancient yogic text, *Yoga Tārāvalī*, Ācārya Śaṅkara described the method of *yoga-nidrā* as:

विच्छिन्नसंकल्पविकल्पमूले निःशेषनिर्मूलितकर्मजाले।
निरन्तराभ्यासनितान्तभद्रा सा जृम्भते योगिनि योगनिद्रा।।२५।।

vicchinna saṁkalpa vikalpa mūle, niḥśeṣa nirmūrita karmajale ।
nirantarābhyāsa nitānta bhadrā sā jṛmbhte yoginī yoga-nidrā ।।
— *Yoga Tārāvalī* 25

When mind has transcended *māyā* (delusion), when ego has become static, when senses are no more functioning, and when all communications between the mind and the senses have been cut, when I and you no longer exist for a period of time *yoga-nidrā* starts.

For a long-time practice, when being disappointed from every resolve and imagination and every obstacle of *karma* becomes destroyed, the *yogī* gets the state of *yoga-nidrā*.

The author of *Haṭha-Yoga Pradīpikā*, great *yogī* Svātmārāma classifies *yoga-nidrā* as the state of *turīya*; means the all expansive and encompassing "fourth dimension" in which Śakti neither contracts nor expands, but is in union with Śiva or the supreme consciousness.

अभ्यसेत् खेचरीं तावद्यावत् स्याद्योगनिद्रितः।
संप्राप्तयोगनिद्रस्य कालो नास्ति कदाचन।।४९।।

abhyaset khecharīṁ tāvadyāvat syādyoganidritaḥ ।
saṁprāpta yoga-nidrā sya kālo nāsti kadācana ।।
— *Haṭha-Yoga Pradīpikā* 4.49

Khecarī should be practised until yogic sleep occurs. For one who has attained yogic sleep, time becomes non-existent. Here the term *yoga-nidrā* has used as the state of *samādhi*. Yogic sleep *(yoga-nidrā)* is the state in which conscious mind subsides but awareness remains.

3

Yoga-Nidrā in Relation to Sleep

SLEEP is one of the greatest inventions of nature and a blessing in life. It is a periodic rest of the body which is absolutely essential for its efficient functioning, it has been called "most cheering restorative of tired bodies". It is the indispensable condition to the recuperation of energy. We go to bed fatigued and get up refreshed.

Sleep is a state of unconsciousness in which the brain is relatively more responsive to internal than to external stimuli. The predictable cycling of sleep and the reversal of relative external unresponsiveness are features that assist in distinguishing sleep from other states of unconsciousness. The brain gradually becomes less responsive to visual, auditory and other environmental stimuli during the transition from wake to sleep, which is considered by some as Stage 1 of sleep.

Historically, sleep was thought to be a passive state that was initiated through withdrawal of sensory input. Currently, withdrawal of sensory awareness is believed to be a factor in sleep, but an active initiation mechanism that facilitates brain withdrawal is also recognized.

यत्र सुप्तो न कंचन कामं कामयेत न कंचन स्वप्नं पश्यति तत्सुषुप्तम् ।
सुषुप्तस्थान एकीभूतः प्रज्ञानघन एवानन्दमयो ह्यानन्दभुक् चेतोमुखः
प्राज्ञस्तृतीयः पादः ।।५।।

yatra supto na kañcana kāmaṁ kāmayate na kañcana svapnaṁ paśyati tatsuṣuptam ।
suṣuptasthāna ekībhūtaḥ prajñānaghana evānandmayo hyānanda bhuk cetomukhaḥ prājñastṛtīyaḥ pādaḥ ।।

— *Māṇḍūkyopaniṣad* 5

In the *Māṇḍūkyopaniṣad* sleep is defined as *prajñā,* where the knowledge, awareness or consciousness are withdrawn into the state of unconsciousness; where the consciousness doesn't extend beyond its boundaries or interact with any of the external series whether physical or mental; theist state of *prajñā* is awareness of the one without a second, "the state of non-duality". The *Māṇḍūkya Upaniṣad* further states that this state of *nidrā* is similar to the state of *samādhi* for the same region. The only difference is that, in *nidrā* there is total introversion with sensory and mental blockage, whereas in *samādhi* there is no total introversion, the mind is alert and awake. Yet it is contained within itself.

The *Yoga-Sūtras* gives a precise definition of *nidrā* as: अभावप्रत्ययालम्बना वृत्तिर्निद्रा॥१०॥ *abhāva pratyālambana vr̥ttir nidrā* (*Pātañjala Yoga-Sūtras* I.10), the state of mind in which its (extrovert) tendency to experience the gross material existence disappears. In the state of *nidrā* the perception of the outside world is introverted and there is sensory, external blockage. The perceptions of the external environment of the body and mind are not recognized consciously or unconsciously. The sleep that the *Yoga-Sūtras* talks about is not the state of dream. It is deep sleep where there is no vacillation and no experience of any kind of mental faculty.

Nidrā is known as *vr̥tti,* because there is no awareness in *nidrā,* and this lack of awareness creates a disturbance in the pattern of consciousness, of mind experience. This lack of awareness does not give the feeling the knowledge or the understanding of time–space and object. This state of deep introversion is a spontaneous withdrawal of the externalized mind, it is not voluntary. In meditation there is voluntary introversion where there is awareness of the different states of experience, while in sleep there is no voluntary introversion, it comes as a natural state.

Sleep is very nicely defined in the Ayurvedic text *Caraka Saṁhitā* as:

यदा तु मनसि क्लान्ते कर्मात्मानः क्लमान्विताः।
विषयेभ्यो निवर्तन्ते तदा स्वपिति मानवः॥

yadā tu manasi klānte karmātmānaḥ klamānvitāḥ ।
viṣayebhyo nivartante tadā svapiti mānavaḥ ॥
— *Caraka Saṁhitā* 21.35

When due to tired mind, the tired entire body senses repel from their series objects, the man falls into sleep. Sleep is a state when the entire body senses in conjugation of *manas* (mind) get detached from their objects.

Let's Define Sleep

Sleep is a physical and mental resting state in which a person becomes relatively inactive and unaware of the environment. In essence, sleep is a partial detachment from the world, where most external stimuli are blocked from the senses.

Normal sleep is characterized by a general decrease in body temperature, blood pressure, breathing rate and most other bodily functions. In contrast, the human brain never decreases its activity. Studies have shown that the brain is as active during sleep as it is when awake. Throughout an eight-hour sleep cycle, a normal adult alternates between two very different states — non-REM and REM (Rapid Eye Movement) sleep.

Sleep Cycle

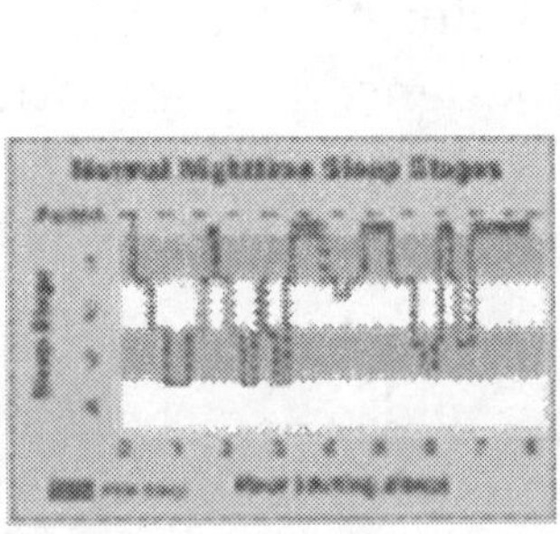

Non-REM sleep and REM sleep alternate in 90-110 minute cycles. A normal sleep pattern has 4-5 cycles. The diagram and descriptions below illustrate the architecture of sleep. This explains why the cycles of sleep have been compared to going up and down a stairway.

The five-step sleep cycle repeats itself throughout a night of sleeping, much like a roller coaster. As a person drifts off, Stage 1 begins. After a few minutes, the electroencephalogram (EEG) detects sleep. It may take anywhere from 30-40 minutes to cycle through Stage 2 through Stage 4. Now, an individual backtracks through Stage 3, then Stage 2, and finally into REM sleep. This occurs 4-5 times per night.

NON-REM SLEEP

Non-REM sleep consists of four stages that range from light dozing to deep sleep. Throughout this state of sleep, muscle activity is still functional, breathing is low and the brain activity is minimal. Approximately 75 per cent of the sleep cycle is spent in non-REM sleep. Simple thought processes may be reported if a person is awakened in any stage of non-REM sleep; however, he or she will not usually recall any specific dream.

Wakefulness: This is a state of awareness in which an individual is conscious of his or her surrounding environment and has the ability to interact with it. In the period before sleep, wakefulness is described as quiet wakefulness, where the individual is resting in a relaxed condition with his or her eyes closed. This stage is characterized by alpha and beta waves activity. Wakefulness is characterized by fast, low voltage EEG activity with both alpha and beta waves present.

Stage 1: This stage could be termed the "dozing" stage. Only 5 per cent of non-REM sleep is spent in Stage 1. It is the transitional period of very light sleep. Although the muscles and breathing rate begin to relax, the individual can still be awakened easily. It is during this stage that, often, a sleeping individual may experience the sensation of falling and jerk suddenly into wakefulness. This is called a hyping jerk. After this rush of activity subsides, the body begins to drift into a light slumber.

Stage 1 sleep is a transition period from wakefulness to sleep. It is characterized by low voltage EEG and slow rolling eye movements.

Stage 2: This stage is often considered the official onset of consolidated sleep. Approximately 45 per cent of non-REM sleep is spent in Stage 2. Eye movements stop and brain waves become larger. Stage 2 sleep is graphically defined with two distinct brain-wave forms, called sleep spindles and K-complexes. A sleep spindle is a pattern of EEG waves, consisting of a burst of 11-15 Hz waves that last for 0.5 to 1.5 seconds. A K-complex is a high-voltage EEG activity that consists of a sharp downward component followed by a slower upward component and lasts more than 0.5 second.

Stage 2 sleep is characterized by a lack of eye movements, sleep spindles and K-complexes.

Stage 3: As sleep advances progressively deeper, an individual becomes difficult to arouse. A person spends approximately 12 per cent of non-REM sleep in this stage. Actual slow-wave sleep begins as large and slow delta waves intermingle with smaller, faster ones.

This stage of sleep is characterized by 20-40 per cent of slow-wave (delta) sleep. Note the delta waves.

Stage 4: It is characterized by very deep sleep. Of the roughly 75 per cent of non-REM sleep, approximately 13 per cent is spent in this final stage. A person in one of the two latter stages, i.e. stage 3 or 4 is harder to wake than a person in Stage 1 or 2. People who wake during deep sleep often feel groggy and disoriented for several minutes. By the time a person shifts into Stage 4, the brain produces delta waves almost exclusively.

Greater than 50 per cent of Stage 4 sleep is characterized by delta waves. Note that there are few graphical differences between Stage 3 and Stage 4.

REM SLEEP

Most dreaming takes place during REM sleep. Periodic eyelid fluttering, muscle paralysis, and irregular breathing, body temperature, heart rate and blood pressure distinguish REM from non-REM sleep. REM sleep is also called "paradoxical" sleep because brain-wave activity is similar to an awakened state. It is during REM sleep that the brain blocks signals to the muscles to remain immobile so dreams will not be acted out. Adults spend about 20-25 per cent of their sleep cycle in REM sleep. The EEG activity during REM sleep shows mixed frequency and low voltage with occasional bursts of "saw tooth" waves. Compare this EEG pattern with the wakefulness pattern.

What determines when we sleep? A major reason why humans sleep is due to circadian rhythms, also known as the biological clock. A cycle that lasts 24 hours is called circadian. Some physiological functions that are circadian include body temperature and certain hormone secretions. So humans have a natural cycle of approximately the length of one day.

Small structures in the brain, called suprachiasmatic nuclei (SCN) co-ordinate circadian rhythms. SCN, in turn, are very sensitive to the presence or absence of light. This may explain why daytime sleep has been found to be less restful than night-time sleep.

Sleep and wakefulness alternate, usually between night and day, respectively. For most people, sleepy peaks occur every 12 hours, at night, and around mid-afternoon. Through a complex process of hormonal and neurological changes, daylight naturally triggers periods of wakefulness. Studies have shown, however, that the absence of light does not disable our biological clock.

The longer a person stays awake, the more sleep him or she requires; thus, the need to sleep accumulates throughout the time of wakefulness. This regulation is called homeostatic because it allows the body to reverse the effects of sleepiness by sleeping.

Normal peaks of alertness occur during daylight hours. The mid-afternoon dip, called a post-prandial dip (after lunch), is caused by a natural decrease in body temperature. When our body temperature begins to drop, we feel sleepy than when it begins to rise.

Reasons for Sleep

Sleep is not a waste of time. Although researchers are not exactly sure why we need sleep, there are two basic theories.

Restorative sleep. It enables the body and mind to rejuvenate, re-energize and restore. As a person sleeps, it is thought that the brain performs vital housekeeping tasks such as organizing long-term memory, integrating new information, and repairing and renewing tissues, nerve cells and other biochemical functions. Sleep allows the body to rest and the mind to sort out past, present and future activities and feelings.

Adaptive Sleep. It may have evolved as a protective adaptation-finding food in the daytime and hiding at night is easier. Nearly every animal sleeps to some degree. Thus, it only makes sense that predators sleep more than animals that are prey. For humans, the amount and quality of sleep achieved are directly proportional to the amount and quality of the next day's productivity.

WHY IS SLEEP IMPORTANT?

Sleep is a necessary and vital biological function. It is essential to a person's physical and emotional well-being. Studies have shown that without enough sleep, a person's ability to perform even simple tasks declines dramatically.

The average sleep-deprived individual may experience impaired performance, irritability, lack of concentration and daytime drowsiness. They are less alert, attentive and unable to concentrate effectively. Additionally, because sleep is linked to restorative processes in the immune system, sleep deprivation in a normal adult causes a biological response similar to the body fighting off an infection.

Persistent sleep deprivation can cause significant mood swings, erratic behaviour, hallucinations and in the most extreme, yet rare cases, death. The jury is still out on the long-term effects of sleep deprivation on health. Current researches in this area are examining the effects of sleep deprivation on the immune system.

A pioneer in sleep research, William Dement, noted that most undergraduates enter college with some knowledge of personal health, but little to no knowledge of the value of sleep. He suggests that all students should not only learn the importance of physical fitness and good nutrition, but healthy sleep, calling all three the "fundamental triumvirate of health".

Robert A. Baron says that sleep is a process in which important psychological changes (including shifts in brain activity and slowing of basic bodily function) are accompanied by major shifts in consciousness.

Lack of sleep is equally dangerous to the healthy functioning of the conscious and the unconscious mind. Because the conscious mind does not get time to relax without sound sleep.

देहवृत्तौ यथाऽऽहारस्तथा स्वप्नः सुखो मतः।
स्वप्नाहारसमुत्थे च स्थौल्यकार्श्ये विशेषतः॥

deha vr̥ttau yathā ''hārastathā svapnaḥ sukho mataḥ ।
svapnāhārsamutthe ca sthanlyakārśye viśeṣataḥ ॥
— *Caraka Saṁhitā* 21.51

Sleep is a periodic and reversible physiologic state, which is necessary for the repair of organs. During the sleep, consciousness is depressed and threshold of sensory perception is considerably increased, and spontaneous movements and muscle tone are reduced to a minimum, while metabolism and visceral functions are not markedly diminished. This concept of modern physiology fully justifies the definition of sleep propounded by our great seer Maharṣi Caraka.

पुष्टिवर्णबलोत्साहमग्निदीप्तिमतन्द्रिताम्।
करोति धातुसाम्यं च निद्रा काले निषेविता॥८८॥

puṣṭivarṇabalotsāhamagnidīptimatandritām ।
karoti dhātusāmyaṁ ca nidrā kāle niṣevitā ॥
— *Suśruta Saṁhitā*, Cikitsā sthāna, 24.88

According to Maharṣi Suśruta a good sleep enjoyed at the proper time for the proper period tends to improve the growth, strength, vigour and complexion of the body. It increases the power of digestion, removes drowsiness and restores the natural equilibrium among the different body tissues.

WHAT IS SLEEP?

As a person moves from a waking state to deep sleep, complex changes in the electrical activity of the brain occur. These changes can be measured with a precision and the resulting EEG reveals much about the nature of sleep. As an individual falls asleep, the electrical activity of her or his brain changes in an orderly manner.

When someone is fully awake and alert, EEG contains many beta waves: relativity high frequency (14-30 Hz), low voltage activity. As he enters a quite resting state (just after getting into bed for sleep or lying into *śavāsana* for the practice of *yoga-nidrā*), beta waves are replaced by alpha waves: EEG activity is somewhat lower in frequency (8-13 Hz) but slightly higher in voltage. As he begins to fall asleep, alpha waves are replaced by even slower delta waves, reflecting the fact that increasingly large numbers of neurons are firing together, in a synchronized manner.

Mental and physical exertions bring about inactivity of the mind resulting in its dissociation from the sense-organs and thereby with their objects, which is responsible for sleep. If there is excessive excretion, this may cause vitiation of *vāta* leading to sleeplessness. By nature, the night serves as a causative factor for sleep. Whereas sleep during daytime is predominately governed by *tamas* and apart from that there are many other factors which are responsible for sleep.

> तमोभवा श्लेष्मसमुद्भवा च मनःशरीरश्रमसंभवा च।
> आगन्तुकी व्याध्यनुवर्तिनी च रात्रिस्वभावप्रभवा च निद्रा।।५८।।
>
> *tamobhavā śleṣma samuddhavā ca manaḥ śarīrśramasaṁbhavā ca* ।
> *āgantukī vyādhyanuvartinī ca rātri svabhāva prabhvā ca nidrā* ।।
>
> रात्रिस्वभावप्रभवा मता या तां भूतधात्रीं प्रवदन्ति तज्ज्ञाः।
> तमोभवामाहुरघस्य मूलं, शेषः पुनर्व्याधिषु निर्दिशन्ति।।५९।।
>
> *rātri svabhāvaprabhavā matā yā tāṁ bhūtadhātrīṁ pravadanti tajjñāḥ* ।
> *tamobhavāmāhuraghasya mūlaṁ, śeṣaḥ punarvyādhiṣu nirdiśanti* ।।59।।
>
> — *Caraka Saṁhitā* 21.58-59

Maharṣi Caraka has enumerated seven types of sleep:

1. Due to *tamas*
2. Due to *kapha*
3. Due to mental exertion
4. Due to physical exhaustion
5. *Āgantuka* (accidental factors)
6. *Vyādhyānuvartinī* (caused by disease)
7. *Rātri-svabhāva* (physiological sleep caused by nature of night).

Robert A. Baron in his book *Psychology* writes that sleep can be divided into four different stages. The transition from wakefulness to sleep occurs with the onset of Stage 1 sleep. During this stage, a mixed but relatively slow low voltage EEG patterns emerges. Breathing slows, muscle tone decreases and the body generally relaxes. At this point individuals can still be readily awakened by external stimuli.

After that they move into Stage 2. During this stage the brain emits occasional short bursts of rapid high-voltage waves known as sleep spindles. Here the person is much more difficult to awaken than he was during Stage 1. Stages 3 and 4 are marked by the increasing appearance of slow, high-voltage delta waves and by a further slowing of all major bodily functions. About 90 minutes after, more and more deep sleep begins which is a highly distinct phase known as REM sleep. During this phase, the electrical activity of the brain changes rapidly; it now closely resembles that shown when people are awake. Delta waves disappear and fast, low-voltage activity returns. The person begins moving the eyelids rapidly. There is almost total suppression of activity in body muscles. Indeed muscle relaxation is so great that a state bordering on paralysis seems to exist. The duration is variable, but the REM periods tend to increase in length towards morning.

The respiration patterns are found to become irregular in this phase. Breathing might even stop for few seconds, but soon regains the normal phase.

The temperature of brain fluctuates and so does the flow of blood in the cerebrum. The expression of dream, and the functioning of the brain and the body imply that the mind is not asleep in this period.

According to Arun Goel (2001) *yoga-nidrā* is a superlative relaxation tool. One hour of effective *yoga-nidrā* is equivalent to over four hours of sleep. But, the true purpose of *yoga-nidrā* goes well beyond deep relaxation. *Yoga-nidrā* establishes the link between the conscious desires, the will-power, the subconscious and the unconscious mind. When this happens you reap all-round powerful benefits and feel in total control of all aspects of your life.

4

Yoga-Nidrā in Relation to Dream

DREAMS are usually the reflections of our memory and medium of expression of our inner tendencies, aspirations and reflections of the unconscious mind. The latter seems to work beyond the limit of space and time. It may exhume the hidden memories of the past — including even the past lives — and express the same in dreams. At the same time, it may also reflect, as per its natural tendency, the experiences in the present conditions of the mind, body and surroundings.

The whole philosophy of dream is very nicely described in the fourth question and answer in *Praśnopaniṣad* (the talk of Ṛṣi Pippalāda and Ṛṣi Gārgya) as:

भगवन्नेतस्मिन् पुरुषे कानि स्वपन्ति?
कान्यस्मिञ्जाग्रति? कतर एष देवः स्वप्नान् पश्यति?
कस्यैतत्सुखं भवति?
कस्मिन्नु सर्वे संप्रतिष्ठिता भवन्तीति ॥

bhagvannetasmin puruṣe kāni svapanti?
kānyasmiñjāgrati? katara eṣa devaḥ svapnān paśyati?
kasyaitatsukhaṁ bhavati?
kaśminnu sarve saṁpratiṣṭhitā bhavantīti ॥
— *Praśnopaniṣad* 4.1

O lord, tell me about those who sleep, those who awake, those who see the dream and enjoy it and where all these things happen?

तस्मै स होवाच। यथा गार्ग्य मरीचयोऽर्कस्यास्तं गच्छतः सर्वा एतस्मिन् तेजोमण्डल एकीभवन्ति। ताः पुनः पुनरुदयतः प्रचरन्त्येवं ह वै तत् सर्वं परे देवे मनस्येकीभवति। तेन तर्ह्येष पुरुषो न शृणोति, न पश्यति, न

जिघ्रति, न रसयते, न स्पृशते, नाभिवदते, नादत्ते, नानन्दयते, न विसृजते, नेयायते, स्वपितीत्याचक्षते ॥

tasmai ssa hovāca । *yathā gārgya marīcayo'rkasyāstaṁ gacchataḥ sarvā etasmin tejomaṇḍala ekībhavanti* । *tāḥ punaḥ punarudayataḥ pracarantyevaṁ ha vai tat sarvaṁ pare deve manasyekībhavati* । *tena tarhyeṣa puruṣo na sr̥ṇoti, na paśyati, na jighrati, na rasayate, na spr̥śate, nābhivadate, nādatte, nānandayate, na viśr̥jate, neyāyate, svapitī-tyācakṣate*

— *Praśnopaniṣad* 4.2

He (Maharṣi Pippalāda) replies to him (Gārgya R̥ṣi). O Gārgya, as during sunset all the sunshine and energy become one, like same during the deep sleep all the sense organs unite with *manas*, and so the person taking sleep doesn't hear; doesn't look; doesn't taste; doesn't touch; doesn't speak; doesn't take; doesn't experience the sex; doesn't excrete and doesn't walk; he sleeps only it has been said.

प्राणाग्नय एवैतस्मिन् पुरे जाग्रति। गार्हपत्यो ह वा एषोऽपानो व्यानोऽन्वाहार्यपचनो यद्गार्हपत्यात् प्रणीयते प्रणयनादाहवनीयः प्राणः

prāṇāgnaya evaitasmin pure jāgrati, gārhapatyo ha vā eṣo 'pāno vyāno 'nvāhāryapacano yadgārhapatyāt praṇīyate praṇayanādāhavanīyaḥ prāṇaḥ ॥ — *Praśnopaniṣad* 4.3

Further he (Maharṣi Pippalāda) expresses: In the city of this body, *agnis* (the subtle fire) of live kinds live in the form of five *prāṇas* and these five *prāṇas* are awake during sleep.

यदुच्छ्वासनिःश्वासावेतावाहुती समं नयतीति स समानः। मनो ह वाव यजमान इष्टफलमेवोदानः स एनं यजमानमहरहर्ब्रह्म गमयति॥

yaducchvāsa-niḥśvāsāvetāvāhutī samaṁ nayatīti sa samānaḥ । *mano ha vāva yajamāna iṣṭaphalamevodānaḥ sa enaṁ yajamānam-aharaharbrahma gamayati* ॥

— *Praśnopaniṣad* 4.4

Here in both these *ślokas* *maharṣi* explains the sleep as *yajana* and the initiation and explanation of breathings are the sacrificing material in the *kuṇḍa* (pit of *yajana*). Through this sacrificing matter the energy is being distributed to the whole body by *samāna vāyu.*

He is the sacrifire (*hotā*) and the *manas* is the performer: *udāna vāyu* is the result of this *karma* who *udāna* brings the performer to *Brahmaloka* or the centre of heart.

In an answer to who dreams, Maharṣi says:

अत्रैष देवः स्वप्ने महिमानमनुभवति। यद् दृष्टं दृष्टमनुपश्यति; श्रुतं श्रुतमेवार्थमनुश्रृणोति; देशदिगन्तरैश्च प्रत्यनुभूतं पुनः पुनः प्रत्यनुभवति; दृष्टं चादृष्टं च, श्रुतं चाश्रुतं चानुभूतं चानुभूतं च, सच्चासच्च, सर्व पश्यति सर्वः पश्यति ॥

atraiṣa devaḥ svapne mahimānamanubhavati। yad dṛṣṭaṁ dṛṣṭamanupaśyati; śrutaṁ śrutamevārthamanuśṛṇoti; deśa-diganta-raiśca pratyanubhūtaṁ punaḥ punaḥ pratyanubhavati; dṛṣṭaṁ cādṛṣṭaṁ ca, śrutaṁ cāśrutaṁ cānubhūtaṁ cānanubhūtaṁ ca, saccāsacca, sarvaṁ paśyati sarvaḥ paśyati ॥ — *Praśnopaniṣad* 4.5

During this state of dream the person experiences all his potential and strength. Here he repeats all the past knowledges like all the visual things he looks; all the heard things he listens and experiences the experienced things again and again. He dreams the new things also but very much related to the circumstances he had experienced already. He *jīvātmā* himself experiences all these.

स यदा तेजसाभिभूतो भवति, अत्रैष देवः स्वप्नान् न पश्यत्यथ तदैतस्मिञ्छरीरे एतत्सुखं भवति ॥

sa yadā tejasābhibhūto bhavati, atraiṣa devaḥ svapnān na paśyatyatha tadaitasmiñcharīre etatsukhaṁ bhavati ॥

— *Praśnopaniṣad* 4.6

During the state of sleep, the *jīvātmā*'s (the person who sleeps) all senses are withdrawn; the *manas* experiences all the dreams and gives the pleasure of dream to the individual.

In brief, *nidrā* is a *yajña* (sacred sacrificial fire) performed in the *kuṇḍa* (pit) of the body where the *pañcāgni*s (five streams of fire) are kindled in the form of the *pañca prāṇa*s (five subliminal currents of vital energy). Breathing is the source of sacrifices made in this *yajña*. The force, which regulates the harmonious flow of vital power in these sacrifices, is the *hotā* (performer) of this *yajña*. Unperturbed cycle of this *yajña* in ones lifetime bestows the fruit of sleep on the mind through the subliminal currents of the *udāna prāṇa*. The *udāna prāṇa* activates the inner (unconscious) cores of mind. Dream is a channel for communicating with the soul and for reaching the *Brahmaloka* — the ultimate realm of the supreme consciousness.

The *Māṇḍūkyopaniṣad* conveys the four stages of consciousness i.e. *jāgrati* (awakened), *suṣupti* (sleep), *svapna* (dream) and *turīya* (bliss). The state of dream is the subtle world of *paramātman* which is in between awakened and sleep states of consciousness.

स्वप्नस्थानस्तैजस उकारो द्वितीया मात्रोत्कर्षादुभयत्वाद्वा उत्कर्षति ह वै ज्ञानसन्ततिं समानश्च भवति नास्याब्रह्मवित्कुले भवति य एवं वेद ।।१०।।

svapnasthānastaijasa ukāro dvitīyā, mātrā utkarṣādu-bhayatvādvā utkarṣati ha vai jñānasantatiṁ samānaśca bhavati nāsyābrahmavitkule bhavati ya evaṁ veda ।।

— *Māṇḍūkyopaniṣad* 10

In this state, the soul can experience the subtle world as naturally as the body feels the physical world. Dream represents an intermediate stage between the awakened and total dormant phase.

Maharṣi Vasiṣṭha had a different view on *svapna* (dream):

इदंजाग्रदयंस्वप्नइतिनास्त्येवभिन्नता।।
सत्येवस्तुनिनिःशेषसमयोर्यानुभूतितः।।२४।।

idaṁ jāgra dayaṁ svapna, iti nāsyeva bhinnatā ।
satye vastūni niḥśeṣa samayoryānubhūtitaḥ ।।

— *Yo.Vā.* 6.2.161.24

There is no difference between the awakened and the dreaming states. The flow of the impulses of the unconscious mind generates dreams. The awakened state too is a dreaming state for soul. In both the states, the soul remains the same.

According to Sigmund Freud dreams provide an important means of probing the unconscious all the thought, impulses and wishes that lie outside the realm of conscious experience. One can give expression to impulses and desires which is unacceptable during the waking hours. In other words, dreams merely represent efforts by our cognitive system to make sense out of this neural activity.

According to a model proposed by Antrobus (1991), dreams occur because during REM sleep, areas of the brain that play a key role in waking perception and thought are highly active while at the same time there is massive inhibition of input from sensory systems and muscles. As a result, the cortical systems that normally regulate perception and thought have only their own output as input. The interpretation of this activity forms the basis for dream.

Dreams appear to be the mode of transmitting subtle messages of the mind through a rhetorically coded language. What everyone sees in the dream is a reflection of the subconscious or unconscious mind. The active dreams of special kind are expressions of the thoughts, sentimental currents and bodily functions in general. The implicit nature of these reflections mingled with multiple flashes of memory makes it almost impossible to decode the meaning of dreams in general. Most often there may not be anything substantial in a dream. The extrovert ambitions and agile mind of people frequently present them with abrupt dreams that are no better than a child's play or conjugation of delusion and arbitrary imaginations.

Modern psychoanalysts of dreams classify them as (a) active and (b) stationary or dull dreams. The first category is attributed to the dreams in which one finds himself as engaged in some activity or as part of a dynamic scene of the dream. The dreamer is merely a silent onlooker of the stationary dreams; one is not a part or an actor in such a dream. Stationary dreams may sometimes inspire a new thought or flash out a novel idea in the viewer's mind. Dreams of this kind also allay mental tension and stress, and soothe the nerves.

Acharya Sri Ram Sharma writes in his book *Sleep Dream and Spiritual Reflections* (pp. 8-9):

> Dreams are termed as mirrors reflecting the basic nature and intrinsic tendencies of the individual self. The nature of one's dreams helps inferring his psychology to some extent. Especially, the roots of intensive influence of fear, lust, ferociousness, aversion, etc., in one's mind are easily diagnosed by decipheration of his dreams.

Dreams are simply our subjective experience of what is, in essence, random neural activity in the brain such activity may reflect ongoing information-processing tasks or may occur simply because a minimal amount of stimulation is necessary for the normal functioning of the brain and nervous system.

The vital energy required for the brain functions during dream is negligible as compared to the positive returns in terms of reducing the pressures of untoward impressions registered in the subconscious mind. Similarly during *yoga-nidrā,* the requirement of energy in the body and brain is less than what is required during the awake state of mind.

5

Yoga-Nidrā in Relation to Samādhi

Samādhi is sublime equanimity. There are many wrong notions about *samādhi*. According to some authors, *samādhi* is a state where one's body becomes petrified and looks like a stone. The pulse rate slows down and the metabolic process stops. Suspended animation is the greatest science which has been mastered and perfected by Indian *yogīs*, but it is not *samādhi*. In the state of suspended animation (*jaḍa samādhi*) there is no awareness or knowledge. The stock of subconscious or subliminal impressions remains unexhausted and dormant.

Samādhi does not merely mean a state of steady posture and total unconsciousness. A person who has been able to make the conscious and subconscious forces dormant is really commendable, but that has nothing to do with *yoga* and the ordinary person. If the state does not exhaust muscular, emotional and mental tensions, if it does not bestow peace, power and enlightenment, if it does not remove your complexes, conflicts, schizophrenia, psychological disorders, etc., it is not *samādhi*.

Samādhi has been rightly regarded as a consummation to be wished for devoutly. But we are not to consider *samādhi* merely as a *kriyā* (action). We have to attain perennial *samādhi* and personify it. Ours should be what Kabīr called *sahaja samādhi*, effortless and felicitous *samādhi*. In the state of *sahaja samādhi*, we attain and retain all the *sthitaprajña* qualities described by Lord Kṛṣṇa in the *Bhagavad-Gītā*.

Modern man has developed many scientific superstitions and you have to do away with them. Each and every idea finds currency with us without proper examination. Accept *yoga* in your daily life. *Yoga* is a way of life, a culture of tomorrow. It is not necessary to go to a temple or meditate on your deity, but wherever and whatever you perceive, perceive with sublime equanimity.

Samādhi literary means union (here union means union of individual consciousness and the superconsciousness). The ultimate goal of *yoga* is *samādhi*, nothing else. It is the supreme state of mind as described in *Kaṭhopaniṣad*:

यदा पञ्चावतिष्ठन्ते ज्ञानानि मनसा सह ।
बुद्धिश्च न विचेष्ठति तामाहुः परमां गतिम् ॥

yadā pañcāvatīṣṭhante jñānāni manasā saha ।
buddhiśca na viceṣṭhati tāmāhuḥ paramāṁ gatim ॥
— (ch. 2, vallī 5, v. 10)

When the five senses of perception, together with the mind, are at rest, when the intellect has ceased to function, that, says the sage, is the supreme state, i.e. *samādhi*.

The *Amr̥tanādopaniṣad* gives the six steps of *yoga* including *samādhi*. According to the text, through the entire materialistic thing becomes meaningless is the state of *samādhi*. The *Jābāla Darśanopaniṣad* states that the awakening of *paramātman* and *jīvātman* is only *samādhi* (chapter 10).

Maharṣi Vasiṣṭha states in *Yogavāsiṣṭha*, *samādhi* as a unique method to rest the mind because in the stage of *nirvikalpa samādhi* the practitioner gets the *ātmapada* (self-state) like the unbreakable and a sweet sleep where mind becomes fully calm.

The most effective description of *samādhi* is given in the ancient yogic text the *Yogacūḍāmaṇyopaniṣad*, which states that (protected) rounds of *prāṇāyāma* lead to *pratyāhāra*, twelve (extended durations of) *pratyāhāra*s lead to *dhāraṇā* and twelve such *dhāraṇā*s lead to *dhyāna*. And, twelve *dhyāna*s result in *samādhi*.

Samādhi is the experience of that which exists beyond temporal experience, which is beyond the influence of nature. It is a timeless state beyond birth, death, beginning and end.

Samādhi starts with total concentration on the object of meditation, with no other thought and no awareness of witness remaining.

According to Patañjali's *Yoga-Sūtras* there are six stages of *samādhi*: *savitarka, nirvitarka, savicāra, nirvicāra, ānanda* and *asmitā*. There are names of very subtle fluctuations taking place before the superior *samādhi* — *nirvikalpa*.

Certain yogic texts have described different forms of *samādhi*, because even in *samādhi* there is progression. According to the tradition there are ten stages of *samādhi* but three others have been included in the view of contemporary *yogīs*, which are equally important.

1. *Nidrā*
2. *Sahaja*
3. *Samprajñāta*
4. *Asamprajñāta*
5. *Savitarka*
6. *Nirvitarka*
7. *Savicāra*
8. *Nirvicāra*
9. *Ānanda*
10. *Asmitā*
11. *Sabīja*
12. *Nirbīja*
13. *Mahā*

Nidrā is the first state of *samādhi* which is experienced every night when we sleep. In this state there is an absence of time, space and object.

Samādhi is very nicely described in the *Bhagavad-Gītā* when the intellect, having been perplexed by hearing the words of scriptures, stands immovable in *samādhi*, than you shall attain self-realization, i.e. this is the state where there is complete absence of both external and internal mental modifications, all that remains is awareness. *Samādhi* brings self-realization.

Ādya Śaṅkarācārya defines *samādhi* in *Yoga-Tārāvalī* as:

सदाशिवोक्तानि सपादलक्षलयावधानानि च सन्तिलोके।
नादानुसन्धानसमाधिमेकं मन्यामहे मान्यतमं लयानाम्।।२।।

sadāśivoktāni sapādalakṣa
layāvadhānāni ca santi loke ।
nādānusandhāna samādhimekaṁ
manyāmahe mānyatamaṁ layānām ।।
— *Yoga Tārāvalī* 2

Lord Śiva instantaneously described the thousands of *laya yoga*s existing in this world. Amongst them all I choose *nādānusandhāna*, enquiry into eternal sound, as the best path to *samādhi.*

Samādhi is a spiritual state of consciousness. There are various kinds of *samādhi*. Among the minor *samādhi*s, *savikalpa samādhi* happens to be the highest. Beyond *savikalpa* the *nirvikalpa samādhi* comes, but there is a great gulf between these two: they are two radically different *samādhi*s. Again, there is something even beyond *nirvikalpa samādhi* called *sahaja samādhi*.

In *savikalpa samādhi*, for a short period of time you lose all human consciousness. In this state the conception of time and space is altogether different. For an hour or two hours you are completely in another world. You see there that almost everything is done. Here in this world there are many desires still unfulfilled in yourself and in others. Millions of desires are not fulfilled and millions of things remain to be done. But when you are in *savikalpa samādhi*, you see that practically everything is done; you have nothing to do. You are only an instrument. If you are used, well and good; otherwise, things are all done. But from *savikalpa samādhi* everybody has to return to ordinary consciousness.

Even in *savikalpa samādhi* there are grades. Just as there are brilliant students and poor students in the same class in a school, in *savikalpa samādhi* some aspirants reach the highest grade, while less aspiring seekers reach a lower rung of the ladder, where everything is not as clear and vivid as on the highest level.

In *savikalpa samādhi* there are thoughts and ideas coming from various places, but they do not affect you. While you are meditating, you remain undisturbed and your inner being functions in a dynamic and confident manner. But when you are a little higher, when you have become one with the soul in *nirvikalpa samādhi,* there will be no ideas or thoughts at all. I am trying to explain it in words, but the consciousness of *nirvikalpa samādhi* can never be adequately explained or expressed. I am trying my best to tell you about this from a very high consciousness, but still my mind is expressing it. But in *nirvikalpa samādhi* there is no mind; there is only infinite peace and bliss. There nature's dance stops, and the knower and the known become one. There you enjoy a supremely divine, all-pervading, self-amorous ecstasy. You become the object of enjoyment, you become the enjoyer and you become the enjoyment itself.

When one enters into *nirvikalpa samādhi,* the first thing the aspirant feels is that the heart is larger than the universe itself. Ordinarily he sees the world around him, and the universe seems infinitely larger than what he is. But this is because the world and the universe are perceived by the limited mind. When someone is in *nirvikalpa samādhi,* he experiences the universe as a tiny dot inside his vast heart.

In *nirvikalpa samādhi* there is infinite bliss. Bliss is a vague word to most people. They hear that there is something called bliss, and some people say that they have experienced it, but most individuals have no first-hand knowledge of it. When you enter into *nirvikalpa samādhi,* however, you not only feel bliss, but actually grow into that bliss.

The third thing you feel in *nirvikalpa samādhi* is power. All the power of all the occultists put together is nothing compared with the power you have in *nirvikalpa samādhi.* But the power that you can take from *samādhi* to utilize on earth is infinitesimal compared with the entirety.

Nirvikalpa samādhi is the highest *samādhi* that most realized spiritual masters attain. It lasts for a few hours or a few days, and then one has to come down. When one comes down, what happens? Very often one forgets his own name and age; one cannot speak or think properly. But through continued practice, gradually one becomes able to come down from *nirvikalpa samādhi* and immediately function in a normal way.

Generally, when one enters into *nirvikalpa samādhi,* one does not want to come back into the world again. If one stays there for eighteen or twenty-one days, there is every possibility that the soul will leave the body for good. There were spiritual masters in the hoary past who attained *nirvikalpa samādhi* and did not come down. They attained their highest *samādhi,* but found it impossible to enter into the world atmosphere again and work like human beings. One cannot operate in the world while in that state of consciousness; it is simply impossible. But there is a divine dispensation. If the supreme wants a particular soul to work here on earth, even after twenty-one or twenty-two days, the supreme can take that individual into another channel of dynamic, divine consciousness and have him return to the earth-plane to act. *Sahaja samādhi* is by far the highest type of *samādhi.* In this *samādhi* one is in the highest consciousness but, at the same time, one is able to work in the gross physical world. One maintains the experience of *nirvikalpa samādhi* while simultaneously entering into earthly activities. One has become the soul and, at the same time, is utilizing the body as a perfect instrument. In *sahaja samādhi* one does the usual things that an ordinary human being does. But in the inmost recesses of the heart one is surcharged with divine illumination. When one has this *sahaja samādhi,* one becomes the lord and master of reality. One can go at his sweet will to the highest and then come down to the earth-consciousness to manifest.

Even after achieving the highest type of realization, on very rare occasion, is anyone blessed with *sahaja samādhi*? Very few spiritual masters have achieved this state. For *sahaja samādhi*, the supreme's infinite grace is required. *Sahaja samādhi* comes only when one has established inseparable oneness with the supreme or when one wants to show, on rare occasions, that he is the supreme. He who has achieved *sahaja samādhi* and remains in this *samādhi*, consciously and perfectly manifests god at every second, and is thus the greatest pride of the transcendental supreme.

The word *samādhi* doesn't indicate liberation but is a field of awareness comprising supraconsciousness. It is the result of total one-pointedness of mind and expansion of consciousness from the mundane perception to that of cosmic awareness. It is the final experience of every human being and that which we are all evolving towards.

Just as scientists have developed the means to release nuclear energy from the uranium atom, the *yogī*s found the scientific system to release the energy and consciousness from the *bindu* within the body.

Haṭharatnāvalī states that "when the mind becomes motionless as a result of (deep) concentration that is called *samādhi*". *Gheraṇḍa Saṁhitā* states that detaching the mind from the body one should make it one with the *paramātman* that is known as *samādhi*, which is not a state of any kind of consciousness. As per *Haṭha-Yoga Pradīpikā*, *samādhi* eliminates death and takes one to the greatest bliss of Brahmā.

"When awareness is separate and distinct from *vṛttis* (mental modifications), when waking, dream, and deep sleep pass like clouds, yet awareness of *ātman* remains, that is the experience of total relaxation. That is why, in Tantra, *yoga-nidrā* is said to be the doorway to *samādhi*!" Even Haṭha-yogic text — *Haṭha-Yoga Pradīpikā* — gives equal importance to *yoga-nidrā* and *samādhi*.

अभ्यसेत् खेचरीं तावद्यावत् स्याद्योगनिद्रितः।

abhyaset khecarīṁ tāvadyāvat syādyoganidritaḥ ।
— *Haṭhayoga Pradīpikā* 4.49

Khecarī should be practised until yogic sleep occurs.

Here the term *yoga-nidrā* has been used as the state of *samādhi.* The relation between *yoga-nidrā* and *samādhi* can be understood as *yoga-nidrā* is the step of *samādhi.*

6

Stages of Consciousness and Yoga-Nidrā

CONSCIOUSNESS can be understood through the word existence; where there is existence there is consciousness. An alert cognitive state, in which one is aware of him or her and the situation, can be defined as consciousness. It is the continuous stream of perceptions of which we are aware from moment to moment — our various cognitive processes such as sleeping, dreaming, concentrating and making decisions. Consciousness may be defined as an awareness of the self and/or the environment.

Awareness, attention, cognition, discrimination, memory, responsiveness, volition are at least some of the definable constituents of the unitary state of consciousness. Consciousness is not attention or memory or anyone of the some individual (including awareness). It is a combination of all of these.

Human consciousness may include consciousness of the self as conscious being. Human consciousness may also include higher levels of organized thinking. Human consciousness may be limited by time and space. Human consciousness may seek the unity of universal consciousness, which may not be limited by time and space. Human consciousness may also seek to universalize itself as the mode of consciousness for all conscious being.

Consciousness may include self-consciousness, i.e. awareness of an individual's own existence as a conscious being. Self-consciousness may include the awareness which individuals have of their own thoughts and feelings.

To understand *yoga-nidrā* it is relevant to discuss few related aspects — the different stages of consciousness, sleep, dream, and *samādhi* and its relation with *yoga-nidrā.*

Yoga-nidrā is one such a wonderful technique, not only for physical or mental relaxation but also for preparing the mind for spiritual discipline. It concerns mainly with *pratyāhāra* (withdrawing senses from sense objects) and *dhāraṇā* (concentration).

It is to be understood that ordinary sleep is not relaxation, for tensions cannot always be resolved completely in ordinary sleep. *Yoga-nidrā* is qualitatively a different relaxation. It is a "sleep" where all the burdens are thrown off to attain more blissful state of awareness, a relaxation much more intense than ordinary sleep.

Colin Wilson suggests at least eight degrees of consciousness — from Level 0 to 7. They are: Level 0: deep sleep; Level 1: dreaming or hypnagogic; Level 2: mere awareness or unresponsive waking state; Level 3: self-awareness that is dull and meaningless; Level 4: passive and reactive, normal consciousness that regards life "as a grim battle"; Level 5: an active, spontaneous, happy consciousness in which life is exciting and interesting; Level 6: a transcendent level where time ceases to exist. Wilson does take note of further levels of consciousness as experienced by mystics but gives no details (level 7 is not explained by him).

V. George Mathew states that consciousness has been defined as awareness of awareness. It has emerged as a field of psychology only in recent times though some of its concerns have their roots in religion, mysticism and occultism. The emergence of the study of consciousness in psychology reflects a change in the mentality of people. Today people are more troubled by existential problems than hysteric symptoms. People are asking questions about self-actualization and the possibility of growth instead of how to get rid of pathological symptoms. Consciousness is also becoming a new approach in psychology, a new way of looking at behaviour, based on systems theory and the holistic method. The study of consciousness emphasizes certain areas like dreams, creativity and supernormal experiences. Consciousness has relevance for all science, as it is related to philosophical issues and the model of man. It is empirical, but open to descriptive, theoretical and insightful understanding. In the twenty-first century, psychology may well be redefined as the study of consciousness and all psychology may be rewritten in that perspective. The study of consciousness may also serve to integrate many areas of psychology and other sciences.

The concept of consciousness arises out of the experience of altered states of consciousness. An alteration in consciousness involves qualitative change in perceptual, cognitive and conative aspects. It involves alteration of mediational processes between stimulus and response. Altered states of consciousness can be induced by overstimulation, sensory deprivation or by altering body chemistry.

Waking and Sleeping

These two states, which are so different, are regularly experienced by everybody everyday. Some people experience a pronounced hypnogogic state in between waking and sleeping and some people get vivid hallucinations during this state.

Dreaming

It involves a state which is physiologically and psychologically different from deep sleep. Lucid dream is a still different mode of functioning where the dreamer has the awareness that he is dreaming. This state is said to be conducive for gaining insight into and awareness of the unconscious and is a technique in mystic training.

Hypnosis

This state is characterized by increased suggestibility and surrender of one's will.

Pathological States

The hysteric trance and schizoid states have been studied as altered states of consciousness using the phenomenological approach.

Orgiastic Trances

This type of trance results from group singing and dancing, often associated with religious ceremonies. These may be psi-conducive states.

Drug-Induced States

The notion of altered states of consciousness evolved originally as a result of the study of subjects who were habituated to drugs like Lysergic acid diethy lamide (LSD). Aldous Huxley's *Doors of Perception* which he wrote on the basis of his experiences with Mescaline is one of the pioneering classics in this area. Many of the effects are due to physiological changes like hypoglycemia. Some of the positive experiences include remembering forgotten painful experiences, ego dissolution, seeing beauty and significance in trivial things, and increase in awareness while those who do not trust get bad trips characterized by terror, panic and suicidal tendencies. Though there seem to be some similarities between drug-induced states, and aesthetic and mystic states, the similarities may only be superficial and the drug may be producing these effects by damaging the brain of a person who may not be ready or mature enough for a transformation of personality required for genuine mystic experiences. Therefore, most authorities do not recommend the use of drugs for altering consciousness though some think that under expert supervision the drugs may play a useful role in efforts to alter states of consciousness. Drugs like *gāñjā,* traditionally used for mystic training, produce memory disorders, decrement in complex psychomotor tasks, lethargy, lack of motivation and lowering of testosterone levels. Some develop psychosis.

Aesthetic State

Many great artists have described sudden changes in consciousness revealing great beauty, which inspired them for creation of works of art. It is almost like a veil falling off from the eyes. Some people regard the aesthetic state as "extraverted" mystic experience, i.e. the projection of the experience of integration within onto the external world.

Mystic State

This is the most important among all the altered states of consciousness. The term mystic is used in the sense of beyond description. This is supposed to be the absolute state of pure consciousness. This involves an alteration of the self-process and freedom from symbolic thinking. At the perceptual level there is unity, the experienced emotion is bliss and at the conative level there is control and self-sufficiency.

Mystics, belonging to different mystic traditions, have different names for this experience. Hindus call this *samādhi*, Buddhists *nirvāṇa*, Sūfīs *fanā*, Christian's *pneuma* and the term used in Zen Buddhism is *satori*. Those experiencing this consider this realization of truth or self-realization. This to some extent overlaps with Maslow's transcendent self-actualization. Fragmentary mystic experiences (peak experiences) have been reported by artists, and spontaneous experiences resembling the mystic experience by people viewing landscapes and during childbirth. The highest mystic experience is supposed to be beyond time and space.

Other States of Consciousness

There seems to be no sharp line of demarcation between feeling states and states of consciousness. A person in a fit of rage functions differently from his normal pattern of behaviour. Fainting may involve alterations in consciousness and effects of isolation may produce alterations in consciousness. Activities like sports may induce peak experience in expert players.

Yoga-nidrā and Transcendental Meditation

Transcendental meditation is a combination of *mantra* and *antarmauna*, which means you go on practising a particular *mantra* and become aware of all that is happening in your mind. In *yoga-nidrā* you do not use a *mantra* at all, but you use your own mind without bringing in anything from outside to influence you. In *yoga-nidrā* you have created a system for yourself, a particular series of practices ranging from fifteen minutes to half an hour. During that period you lead your mind as you would lead your baby or anybody else from one point to the next and the next. So in *yoga-nidrā* you are actually training the mind consciously. You are taking the mind from step to step, from point to point. You are not allowing your mind to run riot, whereas in transcendental meditation you are only practising *mantra* and if your mind is just dissipating, you go on watching it. This is the fundamental difference.

Yoga-nidrā and Psychoanalysis

In *yoga-nidrā* there is virtually no knowledge of the experiences, whereas in psychoanalysis you are aware of each and everything that is happening, but at the same time the problems and complexes are brought to the surface and examined. During *yoga-nidrā* the problems and complexes inherent in the mind are dissolved of their own accord in deep states of relaxation. However, in psychoanalysis it is a very lengthy process and finally nothing is resolved. The purpose is the same, but *yoga-nidrā* is very easy. It is not a very technical and complicated process. Practically everyone can do it after a little training.

Indian *yogīs* and mystics classify the seven states of consciousness differently. They point out that human beings normally experience only three states: sleeping, dreaming and waking. In meditation, fleetingly one can experience *turīya*, literally the fourth state, or transcendental consciousness, commonly known as *samādhi*. When this state coexists and stabilizes with the other three, which is the fifth state, where I-consciousness expands to become cosmic consciousness. The sixth state is god consciousness whereby individual sees god everywhere, in everything. The last is unity consciousness: what is within is also outside — pure consciousness and nothing else is.

7

Yoga-Nidrā and the Views of Authors

THE evils of day-to-day life are deposited in our subconscious mind and in due course they exert a deleterious influence on our mental make-up. Just as our house must be swept daily to keep it tidy, to have a normal personality, we must remove the *saṁskāras*, the mental dirt that accumulates daily in our subconscious mind. *Yoga-nidrā* performs this essential service for us, removing our mental abnormalities and clearing the way to spiritual progress. Swami Satyananda Saraswati (1975) explains *yoga-nidrā* as a state of mind between wakefulness and dream.

When someone practises *yoga-nidrā* he opens the deeper phases of the mind. During the practice of *yoga-nidrā* the consciousness is at different levels. Sometimes it is very close to the senses and at others, it is at a very remote distance. When the consciousness is at a remote distance, it is only possible to understand it through the auditory channels. During *yoga-nidrā* the consciousness is suspended for a few moments periodically, which means that it alternates between the subconscious and unconscious states.

For the practice of *yoga-nidrā* one should lie flat on his back and follow the spoken instruction of the *yoga* instructor. It is convenient to use *yoga-nidrā* tape. During the practice there should be no movement by the practitioner, as well as he should try to remain awake and aware of every given instruction.

Swami Satyananda Saraswati has divided the practice of *yoga-nidrā* in six phases: preparation, *saṅkalpa,* body part awareness, breath awareness, feeling and sensation, visualization, and ending of the practice.

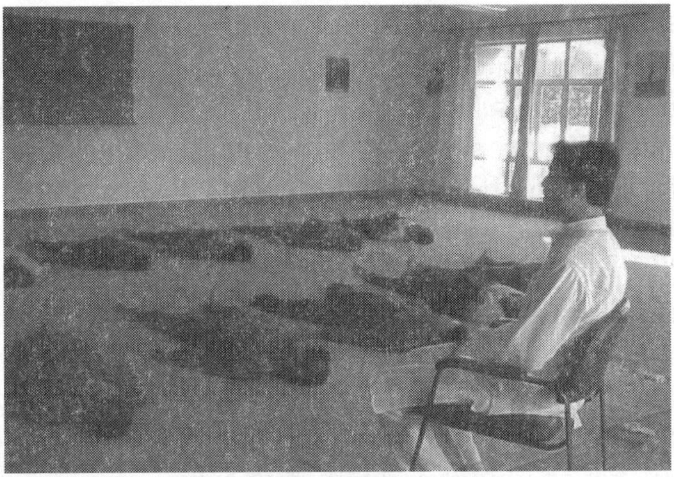

fig. 7.1: Yoga-Nidrā Practice

Preparation for the Practice

Yoga-nidrā is performed in *śavāsana,* which minimizes touch sensation by eliminating contact between the limbs of the body. Fingertips, which are extremely sensitive organs of touch, are kept away from the floor by turning of palms of hands upwards. Light, and loose clothing should be adopted and there should not be breezes of drafts directed towards the body. Sight stimuli are blocked by simply closing the eyes.

The mind is then focused on external sounds. If all sensory impressions are forcibly excluded, then the mind would become restless and disturbed. Therefore the mind is directed to think of external sounds and to move from sound to sound with the attitude of a witness. After some time the mind loses interest in the external world and automatically becomes quiet. This method of calming the mind is called *antarmauna*. It prepares the consciousness for the practice of *yoga-nidrā.*

Saṅkalpa (Resolve)

The Sanskrit word *saṅkalpa* can be translated as "resolve" or "resolution". It is an important technique and a stage of *yoga-nidrā,* and a powerful method of reshaping one's personality along positive lines. To successfully utilize the power of *saṅkalpa* in *yoga-nidrā* one should follow the rules below.

When the body and mind are relaxed, only then the practitioner is instructed to take a resolve according to his or her own wish. The *saṅkalpa* should be short, clear and positive. The practitioner repeats the selected *saṅkalpa* three times mentally, with full determination, conviction and confidence.

Rotation of Consciousness

In the third stage, the awareness is rotated around different body parts in a systematic and organized manner. The practitioner is instructed to remain aware, to listen to the instructions and to move the mind very rapidly according to the instructions without making any physical movements. The rotation of awareness in *yoga-nidrā* follows a definite sequence: right side of the body, beginning with the right hand thumb and ending with the little toe of the right foot; left side of the body, from the left hand thumb to the little toe of the left foot; back of the body, from the heels to the back of the head; and at last the front of the body, from the forehead and individual facial features to the legs.

Breath Awareness

In this stage, one simply becomes aware of the natural breath without making an attempt to change the flow of the breath. One may become aware of the breath by watching it in the nostrils, chest and abdomen, or in the passage between the navel and the throat. The practitioner becomes aware of each incoming and outgoing breath by counting them mentally.

Opposite Feelings and Sensations

In this stage, the physical or emotional sensations are recalled, intensified and experienced fully. Usually this is practised with pairs of opposite feelings or sensations like heat and cold, heaviness and lightness, pain and pleasure, love and hate, and so on.

Visualization

In the state of visualization, the awareness is taken to the dark space in front of the closed eyes, referred to as *cidākāśa* in yogic terminology. The practitioner is then instructed to visualize some objects, stories or situations in the *cidākāśa*.

Saṅkalpa

Once again the *saṅkalpa,* taken in stage two, is repeated mentally three times in this stage with full dedication, faith and optimism.

Ending the Practice

Before ending the session of *Yoga-nidrā,* slowly the awareness is externalized by asking the practitioner to become aware of the external sounds, objects and persons. They are asked then to slowly move the body parts and to stretch the body.

According to Sri Ram Sharma Acharya (1995) *yoga-nidrā* can be understood as scientific sleep. It is a total practice of *yoga* itself. The practices of *śithilāvasthā, śavāsana, śūnyāvasthā* and *samādhi* are of great importance in conditioning the body and mind, which are the different stages of *yoga-nidrā.*

In usual sleep one does not have any control over his dreams. Autosuggestion is impossible in this case. Supernatural experiences of clairvoyance, vision of the invisible, premonition and intuition are also associated with the dreams of divine (or spiritual) category. Deciphering the realities and mechanisms of such dreams elucidates the possibility that individual consciousness can be connected to the vibrations of the subtle world via the "medium" of dreams. The dormant state of the conscious mind and the active intellect during deep sleep coupled with the charged state of the subconscious and unconscious layers of mind may be linked with the state of mind during deep meditation (*dhyāna dhāraṇā*), *yoga-nidrā* and trance. It is in this state that the inspirations of the inner self can be received by our mind without any obstruction and fluctuation. The spiritual realizations experienced by the *yogī*s in the higher states of trance may be described the most real and vivid kinds of dreams.

The practice of *yoga-nidrā* on the contrary allows one to attain a state of "awakened" sleep. In this state, the body and the external mind (and hence the thought process) are made to sleep as per the order of the inner will. The determination, the will-power of the individual self remain active in this state and endeavour auto-suggestive experience of the power of the unconscious mind and its linkage with the soul.

Yoga-nidrā, according to Swami Rama (1998), is a state between sleep and *samādhi*. It is a half-sleep and half-waking state: it is not a waking state and it is not really a sleep state. *Yoga-nidrā* is a state of conscious sleep in which one can record what is going on. There is a fine demarcation between *yoga-nidrā* and *samādhi*. In *yoga-nidrā* one can record those which he cannot receive in the conscious state. When one cannot register something properly in the waking state, they can go into *yoga-nidrā* to register it. *Yoga-nidrā* is used to develop that wisdom that cannot be developed otherwise. He has divided the practice of *Yoga-nidrā* into three phases. In first phase, lie down in *śavāsana* and do sixty-one-point exercise. In the second phase, there is *śithilīkaraṇa* and in the last phase, breathe awareness with the visualization of different *cakra*s (the different psychic centres of subtle body).

The aspirant learns to analyse or resolve all his desires, thoughts and feelings through the practice of *yoga-nidrā*. He attains a state in which he consciously learns to place his mind in deep rest. *Yoga-nidrā* cannot be translated into any other language, but for the convenience of modern students it is called "yogic sleep" or "sleepless sleep". This is a state of conscious sleep in which the student is in deep sleep and yet remains fully conscious. The *yogī*s use this technique for both sleep and meditation. The quality of rest one receives through this method is entirely different from that which is derived through ordinary sleep.

Yoga-nidrā is a revitalizing exercise that gives total rest to the mind, brain, nervous system, senses and body. Except through meditation and *yoga-nidrā*, one cannot give rest to the totality of the mind. There is no drug and no scientific or physical technique so far discovered that gives rest to the unconscious part of the mind, except the technique of *yoga-nidrā*.

Yoga-nidrā is unlike meditation because in meditation one does not seek conscious awareness of the state of deep sleep. During meditation, one learns to practise a steady and comfortable pose, but in *yoga-nidrā,* the corpse posture alone is recommended. *Yoga-nidrā* supports and strengthens the meditational technique. Deep meditation helps the mind attain one-pointedness, while contemplation leads one to the state of constant awareness.

Yoga-nidrā has immense benefits and can be used for learning the subtleties of life. Only by *yoga-nidrā* one can study how the mind slips to dreaming and then goes to deep sleep, how the conscious mind withdraws itself and goes to the lap of the unconscious. The *yogī*s recall all their *saṁskāra*s, watch them, examine, and even select and reject them according to their needs. Those thought patterns that are disturbing are rejected, and those that are helpful are strengthened. With the help and practice of *yoga-nidrā,* one can go beyond all the levels of the unconsciousness.

In the state of dreamless sleep one experiences unity, in contrast to the diversity of the objects experienced in the waking state. *Yogī*s describe this as a void or a state of purely subjective consciousness that has a blissful quality. The sleeper ordinarily enters this blissful state a few times each night and replenishes oneself, but unfortunately, one is not able to be consciously aware of being in that state, so one does not fully experience its blissful quality.

*Yogī*s, therefore, practise methods for extending self-consciousness into this state. They state that the task of the human being is to become consciously aware of the state of deep sleep, which is the unifier of all manifest states and experiences.

But unless the conscious mind is trained to do so, it cannot recall in the waking state memories from the experience of deep sleep. To progress beyond the three manifest states of consciousness of waking, dreaming and deep sleep, the student must learn to consciously gain access to all those states at will and to realize all three states simultaneously, as well as their unity within him and the universe. To accomplish this, *yogīs* learn to go into a deep state of voluntary sleep, called *yoga-nidrā*, and yet remain fully aware of the environment.

In *yoga-nidrā* the clarity of mind is more profound than in the waking state. Often, due to lack of co-ordination of the functions of mind, the mind is clouded and does not remain fully attentive, but in the state of yogic sleep, the mind remains one-pointed and clear. But the highest joy and perennial happiness are realized when one attains the state beyond, *turīya*.

The finest time to practise *yoga-nidrā* is early in the morning before the sun rises or in the evening after sunset. It should be done when it is dark and there is no strain, stimuli, distraction or noise from outside. In the daytime it is difficult to practise well, but if you want to practise it, then you should make your room dark. Usually *yoga-nidrā* is not done before 3 o'clock in the afternoon. The best time to do *yoga-nidrā* is right after meditation if you are not tired and do not fall asleep easily. This practice should not be used for sleep or for relaxation. It should only be done for *yoga-nidrā*. To learn this method you need to have a definite time set aside so that you can practise at the same time everyday. See that you are protected from noise; a little bit of sound can agitate your nervous system and injure your brain fibres; that is why the quiet time of night is preferred.

In the beginning, you should use ten minutes for this exercise. If you are doing it for more than ten minutes in the beginning, then surely you are not doing *yoga-nidrā* but are only sleeping, because the normal capacity of brain wave relaxation is only ten minutes. Your own mind will remind you of your capacity.

The human personality is composed of habit patterns. If *yoga-nidrā* is practised regularly like the practice of meditation, habit will lead you spontaneously to this state. Otherwise to remain fighting mentally — because you are practising it only occasionally — brings frustration. When you think that it is difficult to practise, then it really becomes difficult. But when you decide and determine to practise, your will-power and determination will lead you to achieve what you want to do.

Yogīs reduce the amount of sleep to two and a half hours and finally to no sleep. Using "sleepless sleep", they go to a state of deep meditation instead of sleep. When meditation becomes your whole life this change naturally occurs.

N.C. Panda (2003) explains *yoga-nidrā* as a scientific discipline — the theory, its psychological basis, its techniques and applications — to reveal its significance as a means of strengthening the body's immune system and preventing and curing diseases and regulating one's life patterns. It involves comparative analyses like that of yogic trance and hypnotic trance and Yoga-Vedānta and Freudian psychologies.

8

Scientific Bases of Yoga-Nidrā

Yoga-nidrā is actually an altered state of consciousness. It is neither sleep nor dream nor is it the state of *samādhi*. Aim of the practice of *yoga-nidrā* for the saints and *ṛṣis* of India were to develop the witness attitude, i.e. being aware of the subconscious and unconscious states and ultimately to enter the state of superconsciousness. The practice of *yoga-nidrā* has a number of benefits. Important among them are radiated below.

Minimizes Tension

In the modern world, the international issue is not poverty, drugs or fear of war; it is tension and only tension. A high percentage of people remains in a state of tension and frustration. This continuous level of tension in the body, mind and emotions predisposes the individual towards psychological and psychosomatic disorders. Modern psychology as well as yogic philosophy believe in three kinds of tension — muscular tensions, emotional tensions and mental tensions — which can be progressively released through the systematic and regular practice of *yoga-nidrā*. Muscular tension results from nervous and endocrinal imbalances. It manifests in the form of stiffness and rigidity in the physical body. In the practice of *yoga-nidrā* the body is progressively relaxed, which in turn releases the accumulated muscular tensions.

In day-to-day life, individuals fail to express their emotions freely and openly. As a result, the emotions are repressed and manifest in the form of emotional tension. In the practice of *yoga-nidrā*, the practitioner slowly moves towards the deeper realms of the mind where he or she confronts the deep-rooted emotional tensions. When the practitioner recognizes these emotional tensions with full awareness and a witnessing attitude, then the repressed emotions are released and the practitioner becomes calm and tranquil.

Due to excessive activity on the mental plane, the mind always remains in a state of arousal, which results in mental tension. Throughout life the mind is fed with negative data. In the practice of *yoga-nidrā*, especially in rotation of consciousness and breath awareness, the mind is relaxed, thereby releasing the mental tensions. In this way, through the regular and sincere practice of *yoga-nidrā*, tensions at the physical, emotional and mental level can be minimized. According to Swami Satyananda (1998), "a single hour of *yoga-nidrā* is as restful as four hours of conventional sleep".

Trains the Mind

The *saṅkalpa* taken in each session of *yoga-nidrā* is perhaps the most effective technique for training the mind. Swami Satyananda (1998) says, "Anything in life can fail you, but not the *saṅkalpa* made during *yoga-nidrā*." The *saṅkalpa* is taken and sowed in the subconscious mind when it is relaxed and receptive. The subconscious mind is very obedient and hence carries out the orders immediately. In *yoga-nidrā*, the *saṅkalpa* trains the subconscious mind, and then the ordinary mind follows the path automatically. The *saṅkalpa* helps in training the mind because it is planted when the mind is relaxed and ready to absorb and accept it. The essential thing is that the resolve should be planted with strong will-power and feeling. Many people make conscious resolves guided by intellect, which rarely bring results. Swami Satyananda (1998) says:

> The *saṅkalpa* taken at the beginning of *yoga-nidrā* is like sowing a seed, and the *saṅkalpa* at the end is like irrigating it. So, the resolve taken in *yoga-nidrā* always brings result, if it is taken sincerely.

Relaxes the Mind

The brain is the linking mediator between the mind, body and emotions. In *yoga-nidrā* intensifying the awareness of the body stimulates the brain. When the awareness is rotated on the different body parts, it not only induces physical relaxation but also clears the nerve pathways to the brain. Each of the body parts has an existing centre in the cerebral white matter, named by researchers as "motor homunculus" or "little man". The sequence of rotation of awareness in *yoga-nidrā* is in accordance with the map in the cerebral white matter of the brain. When the awareness is rotated in the same sequence again and again, it induces a flow of prāṇic energy within the neuronal circuit of the motor homunculus of the brain. This prāṇic flow brings in a subjective experience of relaxation in the brain.

In one of the stages of *yoga-nidrā* a pair of opposite feelings or sensations is intensified again and again in the practitioner. This continuous invocation of opposite feelings or sensations is in accordance with the electrophysiological operating principles of the brain. When a neuron fires, it produces a nerve impulse which is relayed and registered in the brain. But if the same neuron keeps on firing again and again, then its relayed impulse is no longer registered by the brain. Researchers have called this phenomenon "habituation". When the brain becomes accustomed to the stimulus, gradually it becomes relaxed. The state where the brain is completely relaxed results in mental relaxation. Sannyasi Mangalteertham (1998) concluded on the basis of his study that the practice of *yoga-nidrā* brings alpha dominance in the brain, which is characterized by mental relaxation.

Clears Up the Unconscious

From early childhood, we tend to repress many wishes, desires and conflicts. Whenever a situation threatens the ego, the defence mechanisms are called upon and the conflicting situation is repressed or suppressed to the unconscious. All the traumatic experiences, unfulfilled desires and threatening situations are suppressed by the ego to the subconscious and unconscious realms of the mind. In the deeper realms of the mind this conflicting and frustrating matter does not die but remains alive and later manifests in the form of various pathological symptoms. The repressed desires, wishes and situations remain in the form of symbols in the unconscious mind.

During the practice of *yoga-nidrā*, the instructor asks the practitioner to visualize certain symbols and images with a witnessing attitude. If the symbols and images are selected properly, they are in accordance with the symbols of the unconscious. An abstract association is created between the guided imagery and the associated repressed experiences of the unconscious. For example, if the teacher instructs the practitioner to visualize a dog, this may bring out a past traumatic childhood experience in which the practitioner was bitten by a dog. The practitioner observes this associated painful experience with a witnessing attitude, which helps in cutting off the personal identification with the experience. When the personal identification ceases to be cut-off, the painful experience associated with the dog is repressed again. In this way, the practice of visualization brings the unconscious repressed desires, experiences, conflicts and frustrations to the conscious level and then cuts off the personal identification with those experiences. As a result, the unconscious is cleared up.

Awakens Creativity

Several examples from the past indicate that creativity is a characteristic of a relaxed and calm mind. When the mind is totally relaxed, the awareness slowly enters the deeper realms (subconscious and unconscious) of the mind and the person becomes aware of the creative and intuitive faculties. Whether it be Newton or Einstein or Mozart, all made significant and vital contributions in the field of creativity when they allowed themselves to relax deeply enough for the images and forms of their unconscious mind to manifest as solutions to their particular problems. Regular practice of *yoga-nidrā* helps in making a bridge between the conscious and unconscious mind. Slowly one becomes tuned with the unconscious workings and then the power of creativity automatically awakens.

Enhances Memory and Learning Capacity

The present popular method of teaching is classroom teaching using rewards and punishments. This method may be good for the intelligent students but is not beneficial for the dull students because the conscious brain or intellect of these students is incapable of receiving the information directly. The technique of *yoga-nidrā* can be used as an educational tool for such dull children, where the knowledge is transmitted directly into the subconscious mind. The technique of *yoga-nidrā* is helpful in increasing learning and memory capacity. When *yoga-nidrā* is used in education, both hemispheres of the student's brain are involved in learning the subject, whereas in classroom teaching the left hemisphere functions more. In this way, the practice of *yoga-nidrā* involves the total mind in learning.

Ostrander and Schroeder (1973) said that "using the technique of *yoga-nidrā* it was possible to teach a foreign language in one-fifth of the time required by conventional methods". Schoolteachers in several countries are using *yoga-nidrā* to augment the capacities of receptivity and attention, and to awaken the joy of learning in their young students. Flak (1978) reported that techniques such as rotation of awareness and visualization heighten the capacity for relaxation and interest among school children.

Counteracts Stress

Stress is a cognitive or emotional response made by the individual towards any situation, which demands adjustment. When the demands of the situation exceed the ability of the individual, distress results, which may manifest in mental and physical symptoms of abnormality. The practice of *yoga-nidrā* helps in building up the coping ability. The practitioner of *yoga-nidrā* slowly becomes aware of the inherent dormant potentialities and thus prevents himself from becoming a victim of distress. Udupa (1977) suggests that stress-related disorders evolve gradually through four stages. In the first stage, psychological symptoms like anxiety and irritability arise due to over activation of the sympathetic nervous system. The second stage is characterized by related physical symptoms like high blood pressure and increased heart rate. In the third stage, the abnormalities manifest clinically in the organ system. In the last stage, severe symptoms in particular organs appear which need long-term medical management.

Swami Satyananda (1998) has said that *yoga-nidrā* is now prescribed by doctors in many countries both as a preventive and curative therapy in the first three stages of stress-related disease. During stress, the sympathetic nervous system becomes activated due to which the organism adopts the "fight or flight" mechanism. In normal circumstances, the parasympathetic system takes over after the emergency goes. But mostly it has been seen that the sympathetic system remains active most of the time resulting in the experience of distress Selye, H (1974). In *yoga-nidrā* an attempt is made to activate the parasympathetic system, and slowly a balance between the sympathetic and parasympathetic systems is achieved by inducing complete physical, emotional and mental relaxation. In this way, the practice of *yoga-nidrā* counteracts stress. Carrington et al. (1980) concluded that *yoga-nidrā* has its most widespread application as a preventive measure to be practised by healthy, active people as a means of relieving accumulated tensions, increasing stress resistance and overall efficiency, and preventing the development of stress-related diseases.

Manages Psychological Disorders

When the individual fails to adjust to the situation, distress steps in. Some individuals are prone to developing distress due to their unconscious urge to remain tense. When distress continues for a long period, it may result in psychological disorders like neuroses or even psychoses. In the practice of *yoga-nidrā*, the inherent tendency to become tense is rooted out and the individual starts viewing the situation as less demanding. Gersten (1978) said that the practitioner of *yoga-nidrā* becomes his own psychotherapist, recognizing and systematically alleviating his own personal problems and interpersonal difficulties. Matthew (1981) reported that *yoga-nidrā* is a successful therapy for both recent and long-standing psychological disturbances of all kinds, especially high anxiety levels and neurotic behaviour patterns. Bahrke (1979) also concluded on the basis of his study that the practice of yogic relaxation has been found to effectively reduce tension and improve the psychological well-being of sufferers from anxiety. On the basis of a study, Bhushan and Sinha (2001) reported that the practice of *yoga-nidrā* significantly reduces the anxiety and hostility level of the practising subjects. Shealy, R.C. (1998) concluded that *yoga-nidrā* is a successful treatment for insomnia. In this manner, various researches show that the technique of *yoga-nidrā* can be successfully administered to manage various psychological disorders.

Manages Psychosomatic Diseases

When the tensions, conflicts and frustrations of the mind manifest in the form of physical symptoms, those diseases are termed as psychosomatic diseases. *Yoga-nidrā* aims at releasing the suppressed and repressed conflicts from the unconscious, thereby relaxing the mind. When the potent cause (tense mind) of psychosomatic disorders is managed, the disease could also be cured. The practice of various stages of *yoga-nidrā*, like *saṅkalpa*, muscular relaxation, breath awareness and guided imagery, have been found to be a significant and effective mode of therapy for asthmatics (Erskine-Milliss and Schonell 1981). Gupta et al. (1979) reported that eighteen out of twenty-seven asthmatic patients showed improvement in respiratory function and greater freedom of breathing after intensive training in *yoga-nidrā* and 63 per cent had definite relaxation and dilation of the bronchial tubes when tested on a Spiro meter. Jansson (1979) reported that after three weeks of relaxation training, the symptoms of colonic irritability were significantly reduced. In the case of cardiac patients, Cooper and Aygen (1979) reported that *yoga-nidrā* significantly lowered levels of serum cholesterol in cardiac patients. Researches also show that the practice of *yoga-nidrā* lowers the elevated blood pressure levels of hypertensive patients (Datey and Bhagat 1977; Bali 1979). In this way, the practice of *yoga-nidrā* effectively manages various psychosomatic diseases.

Since *yoga-nidrā* works in multiple directions efficiently, it has been proved that it is one of the most powerful therapies of relaxation.

9

Previous Studies on Yoga-Nidrā

Yoga-nidrā is a powerful healing tool and is ubiquitous in *yoga* therapy. This is because it is an ultimate method of inducing profound relaxation and deep rest.

Sankardev Saraswati states that resting the body–mind is the fundamental basis on which true and deep healing takes place. Most people find it extremely difficult to rest deeply, especially when they are ill. Many people will not even take time off from work during an illness because of commitments or because they are so driven. This, in turn, may lead to more complex and difficult situations in managing diseases.

Yoga-nidrā can be applied as both a primary therapeutic tool in certain situations, and as an adjunctive treatment for many acute and chronic physical and psychological disease conditions. These conditions include heart disease, high blood pressure, asthma, diabetes, digestive problems arthritis, other chronic degenerative conditions, and some acute conditions such as cough and cold.

Yoga-nidrā is also particularly useful as a tool to recuperate from exhaustion, to manage stressful situations of all kinds, and to manage pre- and post-surgical conditions.

Yoga-nidrā has two main stages. The first stage induces a relaxed state of body–mind. This stage is common in all *yoga-nidrā* practice. The body has the potential to heal itself but requires the correct conditions to allow healing to proceed. The primary condition required for healing is deep rest. The process of inducing deep rest begins with the use of a positive resolution, a resolve that consciously articulates our desire to heal ourselves. Then rotation of awareness through the parts of the body is performed, which is a simplified form of *nyāsa*. Rotation of awareness creates whole body relaxation. This is followed by awareness of and manipulation of the breath which powerfully relaxes the nervous system and the thinking mind.

The second stage is the use of processes that can either be general healing strategies appropriate for the majority of people, or strategies that are specific to the condition being treated. In specific disease conditions the *yoga* therapist must know about the condition they are dealing with, and must understand its nature and its usual progression. This gives the therapist the understanding required to initiate proper treatment.

The second stage of *yoga-nidrā* may employ tactics and techniques such as specific forms of breathing, and instructions to induce feeling-states that rebalance the basic elements of the body–mind. For example, inducing the feeling of heaviness activates the earth and water elements that may be required when a person is feeling ungrounded or anxious. Inducing lightness activates the air and space elements that may be useful when a person is feeling stuck, heavy or depressed. Techniques that work with feelings of heat and cold, pleasure and pain, and thoughts, including memories, attitudes and held beliefs are also employed.

Another important part of *yoga-nidrā* is the use of visualization to create positive images while placing the awareness on affected parts of the body. Positive awareness injects energy for healing into those parts.

With many approaches the scientific studies have been done in different parts of the world to highlight the effect of *yoga-nidrā* and to establish the scientific facts in this relation. Some of the important studies have been mentioned below.

Cooper and Aygen (1979) in an important study at the University of Tel Aviv (Israel) reported that *yoga-nidrā* significantly lowered levels of serum cholesterol in cardiac patients.

Nespor (1981) stated that the future role of *yoga-nidrā* in coronary care and management regimes appears to be a major one. The value of the practice of yogic relaxation in prevention of cardiovascular disease has been fairly well recognized and accepted.

In another study, which was conducted at the Langley Porter Neuropsychiatry Institute in California, Bali (1979) found a reduction in blood pressure and anxiety levels in hypertensive patients as a result of the practice of *yoga-nidrā* training continued for twelve months.

Matthew (1981) reported that *yoga-nidrā* is a successful therapy for both recent and long-standing psychological disturbances of all kinds, especially high anxiety levels and neurotic behaviour patterns.

Carrington et al. concluded in their work, which was published in a medical magazine in 1980 that *yoga-nidrā* has its widespread application as a preventive measure, to be practised by healthy active people as a means of relieving accumulated tensions, increasing stress resistance and overall of psychosomatic disease.

According to Brownstein and Dembert (1998), an American pilot, with a six-year history of high blood pressure, underwent various treatments without results. Following a six-week programme of *yoga* and relaxation, his blood pressure was normalized, and he regained full flight status. The researchers also pointed out that relaxation also has an advantage over medicine in that it had no side effects, something which can be hazardous for a fighter pilot.

Robert Nilsson (1997-98) stated that researchers have for the first time succeeded in taking pictures of the brain during a meditative deep-relaxation, with as short an exposure time as one minute per photograph. The pictures were taken by one of the most advanced medical research instruments, the PET (Positron Emission Tomography) scanner at the State University Hospital in Copenhagen. The initiators — Hans Lou and Troels Kjćr — were researchers from the Kennedy Institute in Copenhagen.

The measurements show, for the first time, that one can be completely aware in such a deep state, and can consciously experience and control the brain's activity simultaneously. This confirms that meditation is a fourth major state, equal to dreaming, sleeping and wakefulness. The results can therefore be said to be a very important news within this field of research!

Rest

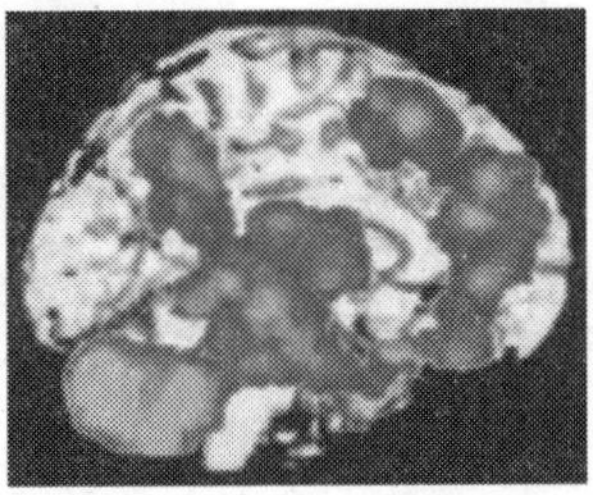

The picture is based on the photographs taken prior to and following *yoga-nidrā*. It illustrates the state closest to normal waking consciousness, though without being a tired or stressed state. Those who use *yoga-nidrā* remark that not only do they get something out of the deep relaxation while doing it, but that it has a definite beneficial effect on the rest of the day.

In the first picture it is the front of the brain that is responsible for the superior control and which is active. One of its capacities is to ensure that we can function in a complex society, as it "processes" the signals from the deeper emotional and instinctive regions of the brain. The brain stem and the cerebellum are also active, indicating that one is "ready for action".

Meditation

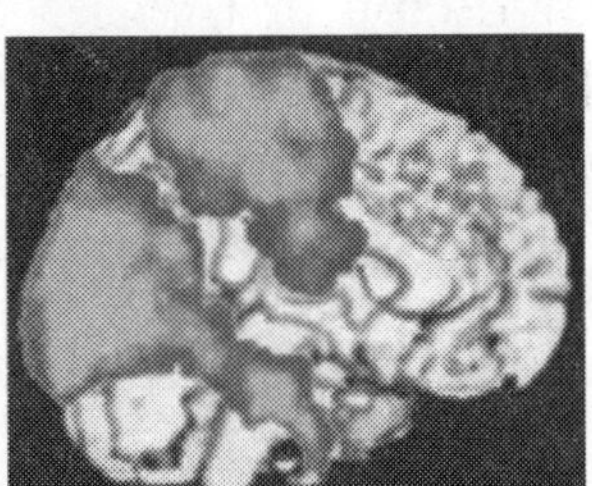

The second picture shows the general state during the entire *yoga-nidrā*. The visual centre at the back of the head and the centre for tactile sense (sense of touch and direction) at the top of the head are active and are in contact with the limbic system. This implies an increased ability to visualize and, more importantly, that there is better contact with emotions.

Some of the teachers also had distinct activity in the centre for long-term memory, which is consistent with accounts from people who meditate, that very lucid memories can appear during or after a meditation.

It must, however, be emphasized from our side that the subjects' experience and their regular use of *kriyā-yoga* possibly intensifies the effects of *yoga-nidrā*.

Abstract

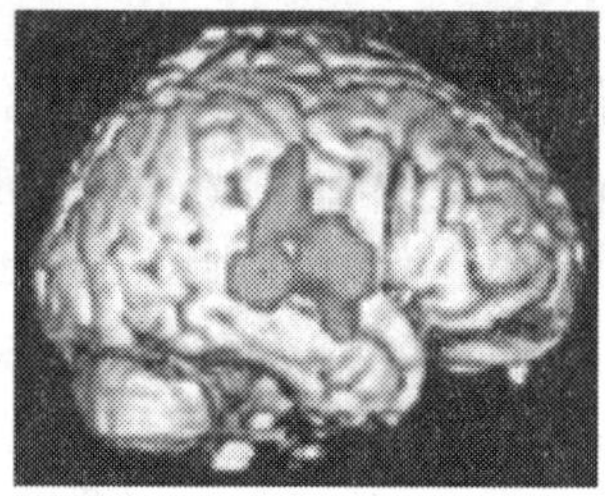

The third picture is created on the basis of measurements taken during the experience of happiness and at the end of the relaxation during the experience of identity, of being centred. During these "abstract experiences" in *yoga-nidrā*, the centre for speech and language was especially active.

It must be said, however, that the pictures only show the areas where the most activity occurs, and not the general activity in the whole brain, as is shown in picture 2.

Concrete

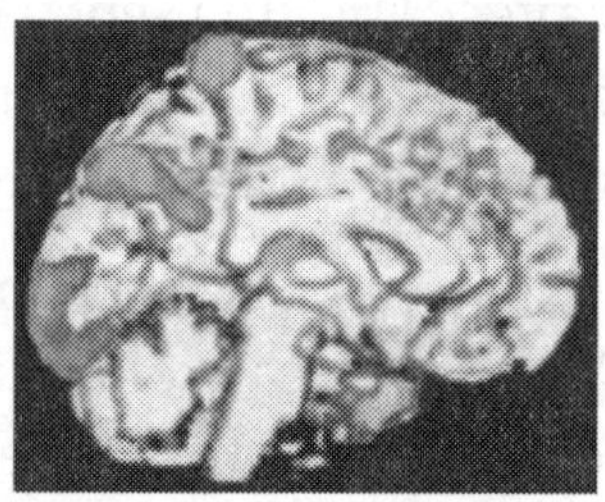

It was primarily the visual and tactile centres which were active as the subjects went through the body's different parts (especially the face) and experienced a pleasant summer day in the country.

When looking at these pictures (1, 2 and 4) one must imagine that the luminous areas are within the brain, and not only on the surface of the cerebral cortex. In picture 3, on the other hand, the activity is in the cortex. All active areas were basically the same, which are symmetrical, in both brain halves.

The pictures of the brain were taken in a PET scanner, which measures the flow of blood through different parts of the brain.

This is done by injecting water with a weak radioactive trace into the blood stream.

According to Sannyasi Mangalteertham (1998), *yoga-nidrā* is probably a best-known technique to induce complete physical, mental and emotional relaxation. This was proved through a series of study done at Cherring Cross Medical School, London, that it is a technique in which one can alter the states of consciousness from beta to alpha and then to delta. Therefore, the subject enjoys the different states of consciousness, knowingly. It is a *pratyāhāra* but also opens the door for meditation. On the basis of his study, he states that the practice of *yoga-nidrā* brings alpha dominance in the brain, which is characterized by mental relaxation.

In another study by Roney-Dougal (2001) initial EEG showed beta activity prominently with intermittent alpha activity. With the advancement of *yoga-nidrā* beta activity was slowly replaced by alpha activity and still further by smooth well-formed alpha activity. After thirty sessions of *yoga-nidrā,* gain of alpha activity was better and with further advancement of *yoga-nidrā* intermittent theta activity was noted intermixed with alpha activity, suggestive of deep state of relaxation. EEG measures minute electrical activity in the brain in the form of waves. The frequency of brain-activity waves has been shown to alter according to the state of consciousness and state of mind the subject is in.

Beta activity is normally noted in the awaken working state. With physical relaxation beta activity is taken up by alpha activity, and as the person goes into different stages of sleep the activity changes to theta and also may exhibit delta activity in deep sleep.

Siddhartha and Sinha (2001) say on the basis of their study that the technique of *yoga-nidrā* has preventive, promotive and curative values. It prevents stress and stress-related disorders by inducing deep physical, emotional and mental relaxation, by training the mind to remain calm and quiet and by rooting out the repressed desires and thoughts from the deeper realms of mind. As a promotive science, *yoga-nidrā* awakens the inherent creativity and promotes the learning and memory abilities of the practitioner. Researches also indicate that *yoga-nidrā* can be used as a therapeutic technique to cure psychological disorders like anxiety, hostility and insomnia, and psychosomatic diseases like asthma, coronary heart disease, cancer and hypertension. In our modern lifestyle, where psychological and psychosomatic problems are on the rise, the technique of *yoga-nidrā* may serve as a real boon for mankind.

Mandlik Yogacharya Vishwas et al. (2002) in their study found that there was psi missing with the preliminary test session.

> At the time it was felt that this was due to the students doing too many preliminary tests, so that they were too rushed and confused by the time the experimental test occurred. Therefore, the students did less preliminary testing, so the less rushed and were more at ease with the procedure. This resulted in improved overall scoring. The relaxation session gives a consistent score over both years. The meditation session compares favourably with the score from the previous year, which was in the psi-hitting range but not significantly so, as does the *yoga-nidrā,* which compares very favourably with the psi-missing of the previous year. This suggests that the lessons learnt from the first year are resulting in an environment, which is more conducive for psi testing. It is, therefore, appropriate now to move from the preliminary exploratory stage to one with proper controls and predetermined statistical analysis.
>
> As not all the students were able to attend each week the participant numbers declined over the four weeks of testing. This needs to be rectified if valid results are to be obtained, particularly with the confounding effect of attitude. The other problem with this design is that it is not counterbalanced, all the students doing the sessions in the same order. It is therefore also possible that there are order effects, the students becoming gradually more accustomed to the procedure, learning from mistakes in previous sessions and so becoming more skilled as the series progressed. A more controlled counterbalanced design is needed if this is to be

rectified and this would need committed participants and splitting the class into at least two groups.

Overall, whilst inconclusive owing to the drop in student numbers and the lack of a counterbalanced design, this year's class research once again suggests that meditation is a psi-conducive state, and there is a possibility that relaxation and *yoga-nidrā* are too. The combined scores from 2002 and 2003 confirm the usefulness of meditation in creating a psi-conducive state of consciousness. In 2002, there was psi-missing with the preliminary test session. At the time it was felt that this was due to the students doing too many preliminary tests, so that they were too rushed and confused by the time the experimental test occurred. Therefore, this year the students did less preliminary testing, so the class was less rushed and they were more at ease with the procedure. This resulted in improved overall scoring. The relaxation session gives a consistent score over both years. The meditation session compares favourably with the score from the previous year, which was in the psi-hitting range but not significantly so, as does the *yoga-nidrā*, which compares very favourably with the psi-missing of the previous year. This suggests that the lessons learnt from the first year are resulting in an environment which is more conducive for psi testing. It is therefore appropriate now to move from the preliminary exploratory stage to one with proper controls and predetermined statistical analysis.

Verma (2004) states on the basis of her study on thirty students for fifteen days practice of *yoga-nidrā* that *yoga-nidrā* has a positive effect in enhancing the memory of children.

Kumar (2004) finds after a six months study on the higher class students that practice of *yoga-nidrā* reduces the stress and anxiety as well as improves the general well-being.

Kumar (2005) observes in another study conducted over primary hypertensive patients for forty days that *yoga-nidrā* affects positively on blood pressure and other psychological co-relates in hypertensive patients.

Kumar (2006) finds in a study on the improvement of

physical and mental health through *yoga-nidrā* that after a six-month study, there is a significant change on the alpha EEG and Galvanic Skin Response (GSR) level of the subjects. This indicates the improvement of physical and mental health as a result of practising *yoga-nidrā*.

Bhushan (2006 a) stated in his study that *yoga-nidrā* can deal with overall personality of a person and it is an effective tool for qualitative transformation in personality.

Deuskar et al. (2006) state that there is a significant effect of *yoga-nidrā* and applied relaxation technique on steadiness and performance of archers.

Bhushan (2006 b) observes in another study that intervention of *yoga-nidrā* can promote self-confidence among teenagers.

Going by the finding of Kumar (2007), *yoga-nidrā* can be considered as a highly effective practice for the practitioners, as it significantly increases the level of haemoglobin of the students at higher classes and there is also an increase in Total Leacocyte Count (TLC) level. Thus *yoga-nidrā* is a complete relaxation process of the body and mind; it increases the immunity of a person, and hence the change in the haemoglobin and TLC is positive. It can be stated that sleep is good for us but present research shows that practising *yoga-nidrā* can not only help us fight off infection, but lower stress level as well.

Pandya and Kumar (2007) state that practice of *yoga-nidrā* is a spiritual technique of total relaxation. They observed a significant change in pulse rate, respiration rate, blood pressure and GSR of the subjects, after a six-month study. They further state that *yoga-nidrā* is able to improve the immunity of the practitioner.

Bhushan (2007) finds the effect of *yoga-nidrā* on qualitative transformation in the personality of youngsters. The study was conducted on two separate samples of eighty-six boys and 102 girls reading in intermediate classes in the two constituent colleges of T.M. Bhagalpur University at Munger. The subjects belonged to the age group of 15-18 years. One hour of *yoga-nidrā* classes were given to the experimental groups continuously for a period of one month while no such practice was given to the control groups. The tridimensional inventory was administered in pre–post condition to measure the level of *sattva, rajas* and *tamas guṇa*s. Comparison of pre–post *yoga-nidrā* period on the selected test indicated that the practice of *yoga-nidrā* substantially increased the level of *sattva guṇa* and significantly decreased the level of *rajas* and *tamas guṇa*s in the practising female subjects in comparison to their control group. Among the male subjects substantial increase in *sattva guṇa* has been found but the decrease in the level of *rajas* and *tamas guṇa*s has not been found significant.

Kumar (2008) observes a significant change in his study in the practice group, result shows that *yoga-nidrā* positively decreases the stress level of the male and female subjects. Several other studies prove that *yoga-nidrā* equally influences anxiety level significantly in both male and female subjects.

Rasal and Deuskar (2008) in their study "Effectiveness of Rational Emotive Therapy (RET) and *Yoga-nidrā* for Anger Management in Families" find that practice of *Yoga-nidrā* helps in family management particularly the anger disorders of the members.

Kumar and Joshi (2009) observe in their study conducted at PG Degree College Haldwani on college-going students that practice of *yoga-nidrā* and *prāṇākarṣaṇa prāṇāyāma* positively increase the alpha EEG and GSR level of the practitioners.

Amita et al. (2009) state in their study that diabetes is a metabolic disorder, which has become a major health challenge worldwide. South-East Asian countries have a highest burden of diabetes. In India the prevalence of diabetes is rising rapidly especially in the urban population because of increasing obesity and reduced physical activity. An objective of this study is to evaluate the effect of *yoga-nidrā* on blood glucose level in diabetic patients.

This study was conducted on forty-one, middle aged, type-2 diabetic patients, who were on oral hypoglycaemic. These patients were divided into two groups: (a) twenty patients on oral hypoglycaemic with *yoga-nidrā*, and (b) twenty-one were on oral hypoglycaemic alone. *Yoga-nidrā* was practised for thirty minutes daily up to ninety days, and parameters were recorded every thirtieth day.

Results of this study show that most of the symptoms were subsided ($P < 0.004$, significant), and fall of mean blood glucose level was significant after three-month of *yoga-nidrā*. This fall was 21.3 mg/dl, $P < 0.0007$ (from 159 ± 12.27 to 137.7 ± 23.15,) in fasting and 17.95 mg/dl, $P = 0.02$ (from 255.45 ± 16.85 to 237.5 ± 30.54) in post-prandial glucose level. Results of this study suggest that subjects on *yoga-nidrā* with drug regimen had better control on fluctuating blood glucose and symptoms associated with diabetes, compared to those on oral hypoglycaemics alone.

Agrawal (2009) concludes through his study that *yoga-nidrā* is one of the effective yogic techniques as an Open Secret of Divine Yogic Self-Healing Technique.

Kumar (2010) opines that *yoga-nidrā* positively decreases the regression and guilt level of the college-going students in both male and female subjects. Several other studies prove the effectiveness of *yoga-nidrā* as well.

Pritchard et al. (2010) observe the effect of *yoga-nidrā* on multiple sclerosis and cancer patients and stated that stress is a common occurrence in many chronically ill patients, and researchers are calling for cost-effective stress-reduction interventions. Meditation techniques have demonstrated a host of benefits for chronically ill patients. The present study examined the effects of a six-week *yoga-nidrā* meditation programme on perceived stress in multiple sclerosis and cancer patients. Overall stress was significantly reduced over the course of the programme.

Rani et al. (2011) observe the impact of *yoga-nidrā* on psychological general well-being in patients with menstrual irregularities and find that patients with menstrual irregularities having psychological problems improved significantly in the areas of their well-being, anxiety and depression by learning and applying a programme based on yogic intervention (*yoga-nidrā*).

Kumar and Pandya (2012) conducted a control-group research study on 110 healthy subjects to observe the impact on ESR level through yogic relaxation technique *yoga-nidrā*. The study shows a significant change on the ESR level of the practice-group subjects as the result of *yoga-nidrā*.

Khushbu Rani et al. (2012) state that emotional insecurity, stress, depressive and/or anxiety symptoms are common with variable severity among patients with menstrual disorder. Yogic relaxation therapy (*yoga-nidrā*) leads to conscious and subconscious recognition of these underlying psychological factors and helps releasing of suppressed conflicts. To evaluate the effect of *yoga-nidrā* on anxiety and depressive symptoms in patients with menstrual disorders subjects were recruited from the Department of Obstetrics and Gynaecology, C.S.M. Medical University (erstwhile KGMU), Lucknow, Uttar Pradesh, India.

The subjects were randomly divided into two groups: intervention group (with yogic intervention) and control group (without yogic intervention). Assessments of all subjects were carried out by administering Hamilton anxiety scale (HAM-A) and Hamilton rating scale for depression (HAM-D) at baseline and after six months. The result showed that there was significant reduction of scores in HAM-A ($P < 0.003$) and HAM-D ($P < 0.02$), respectively, in subjects with mild to moderate anxiety and depressive symptoms after six months of *yoga* therapy (*yoga-nidrā*) in intervention group in comparison to control group. After this study it can be concluded that the patients with mild to moderate anxiety and depressive symptoms improve significantly with *yoga-nidrā* intervention. There is no significant improvement in the patients with severe anxiety and depressive symptoms.

10

Yoga-Nidrā and Human Physiology

It is impossible to ignore the connection between the discoveries of modern brain researchers and those of the enlightened *yogī*s who long ago evolved the practice of *yoga-nidrā*. Of course, the yogic scientists of former ages did not devise this powerful technique merely as a means of alleviating diseases, but primarily as a way of attaining higher consciousness by expanding and liberating individual awareness from its fixation within the physical body and its sensory modalities towards the more subtle "prāṇic", psychic and spiritual dimensions underlying gross material existence.

It is therefore important to investigate multiple aspects of *yoga-nidrā* through interdisciplinary research. The present work applied *yoga-nidrā* in an attempt to investigate the effects of this wonderful yogic practice with multiple dimensions. In this study *yoga-nidrā* has been taken as independent variable whereas some physiological parameters have been taken as dependent variable.

To study the effects of *yoga-nidrā* on some physiological variables we selected the pulse rate, respiration rate and blood pressure.

The pulse rate is normally the number of heartbeats per minute. The resting pulse rate for an average adult is between sixty and eighty beats per minute.

In medicine, a person's pulse is the throbbing of a person's arteries as an effect of his heartbeat, which can be felt at the wrist and other places. The term is also used to denote the frequency of the heartbeat, usually measured in beats per minute. In most people, the pulse is a measure of heart rate, unless some of the heartbeats are ineffective and only displace little blood (as happens in some arrhythmias); in this case, the heart rate can be (much) higher than the pulse.

Respiratory rate is the number of breaths (inspirations and expirations) in one minute. It is the rate of reduction of oxygen concentration due to biological action. The number of breaths per minute, usually measured by movements of the chest.

Sphygmomanometer (with mercury) is the instrument which has been used to measure the blood pressure; blood pressure is the amount of force exerted by the blood against the walls of the arteries. Usually, blood pressure is expressed in two numbers — "diastolic" and "systolic". Diastolic pressure (the bottom number) means the base level of pressure in the arterial system when the heart is momentarily relaxed between beats. "Systolic" pressure (the top number) is the force with which each pulse of blood presses against the arterial walls, as the heart pumps blood out. Such as 120/80 is measured in millimeters of mercury (mm Hg).

Stratified quota sampling was used in this study. The total sample covered for the purpose of the present study belonged to the students of PG Yoga classes from Dev Sanskriti Vishwavidyalaya, Shantikunj, Haridwar; who were of between 20-30 age group and 110 in numbers (fifty-five males and fifty-five females). They were further divided into forty males and forty females in experimental group; as well as fifteen males and fifteen females in control group. In the study, control-group research design was adopted.

To measure the pulse of the subjects, pulse biofeedback was put in application, which is a process of monitoring and displaying to an individual the ongoing heartbeat. Its most common clinical application is to control dangerous heartbeat irregularities by force of mental discipline alone. It is important to control tachycardia and these irregularities or premature ventricular contractions as their presence is associated with an increased probability of sudden death.

In pulse biofeedback, pulse signal is detected by IR transducer, applied on the finger of the person, then amplified, filtered, processed and translated into visual and auditory feedback displays. Pulse rate per minute is also displayed in digital panel meter.

To measure the respiration rate, respiration biofeedback was used which is the biofeedback of the abdominal respiratory excursion. It has been proved to be a psychotherapeutic training method which is easy to apply and which has rapid and intensive effects. The new residual free bubble (rfb)-method confirms the hypothesis of "organismic switching" in autogenic training with a resulting reduction of central nervous arousal during relaxation. To a large extent its psychotherapeutic dimension has been psychometrically and clinically recorded.

By using respiration for biofeedback, rfb's application is more immediate than the self-practice of other relaxation methods. Its focal point is the basic care of patients which is difficult, if not impossible, to read with other psychotherapeutic methods. It can also open up people for conflict-centred psychotherapy.

Hypothesis and Result

HYPOTHESIS 1

The practice of *yoga-nidrā* will decrease the pulse rate of the male subjects.

Table 10.1: Pulse Rate Level of Male Subjects

	Mean	sd	"t" Value	Sig. Level
Experimental	66.87	8.80	3.40	At 0.01
Control	71.53	6.17		

Table 10.1 shows that the post-mean values of the experimental and control groups are 66.87 and 71.53, respectively, and the "t" value is 3.40; a significant change at 0.01 significance level in the pulse rate of the male subjects of

the experimental and control groups; thus Hypothesis 1 has been proved.

HYPOTHESIS 2

The practice of *yoga-nidrā* will decrease the pulse rate of the female subjects.

Table 10.2: Pulse Rate Level of Female Subjects

	Mean	sd	"t" Value	Sig. Level
Experimental	2.62	5.10	5.20	At 0.01
Control	78.13	4.61		

Table 10.2 shows that the post-mean values of the experimental and control groups are 72.62 and 78.13, respectively and the "t" value is 5.20; a significant change at 0.01 significance level in the pulse rate of the female subjects of the experimental and control groups; thus Hypothesis 2 has been proved.

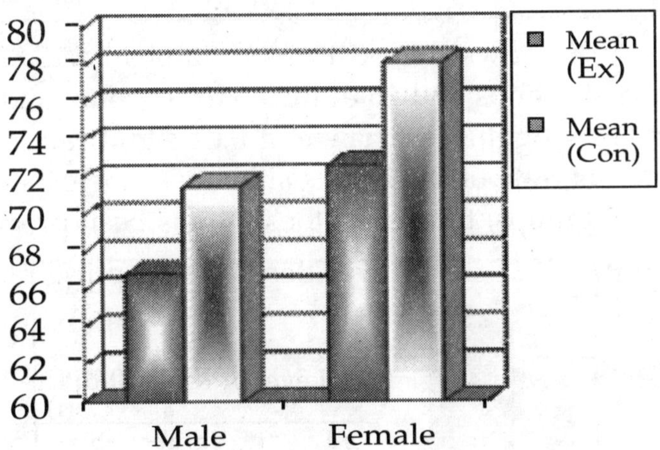

Graph 10.1: Pulse Rate

Graph 10.1 shows the post-values of pulse rate of the experimental and control groups.

HYPOTHESIS 3

The practice of *yoga-nidrā* will decrease the respiration rate of the male subjects.

Table 10.3: Respiratory Rate for Male Subjects

	Mean	sd	"t" Value	Sig. Level
Experimental	14.23	3.75	6.01	At 0.01
Control	7.60	1.35		

Table 10.3 shows the post-mean values as 14.23 of the experimental group and 17.60 of the control group, and the "t" value is 6.01; a significant change at 0.01 significance level in the respiration rate of the male subjects of the experimental and control groups; thus Hypothesis 3 has been proved.

HYPOTHESIS 4

The practice of *yoga-nidrā* will decrease the respiration rate of the female subjects.

Table 10.4: Respiratory Rate for Female Subjects

	Mean	sd	"t" Value	Sig. Level
Experimental	13.82	2.60	4.6	At 0.01
Control	16.00	2.65		

Table 10.4 shows the post-mean values as 13.82 of the experimental groups and 16 of the control group, and the "t" value is 4.6; a significant change at 0.01 significance level in the respiration rate of the female subjects of the experimental and control groups; thus Hypothesis 4 has been proved.

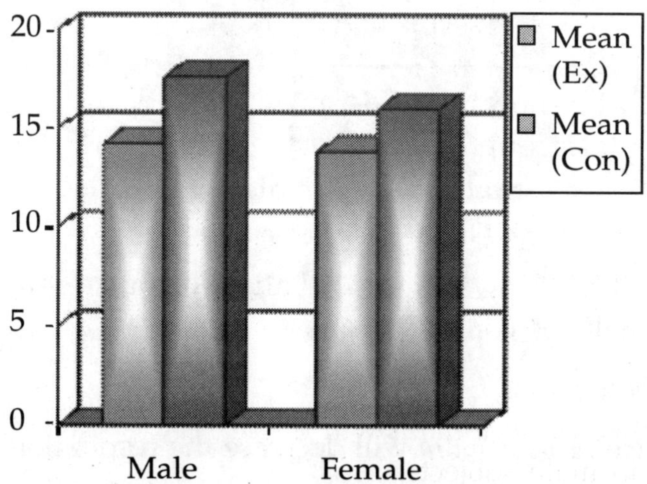

Graph 10.2: Respiration Rate

Graph 10.2 shows the post-values of respiration rate of the experimental and control groups.

HYPOTHESIS 5

The practice of *yoga-nidrā* will decrease the systolic blood pressure in male subjects.

Table 10.5: Systolic BP in Male Subjects

	Mean	sd	"t" Value	Sig. Level
Experimental	111.65	8.82	3.55	At 0.01
Control	117.33	7.99		

Table 10.5 shows the post-mean values as 111.65 of the experimental group and 117.33 of the control group, and the "t" value is 3.55; a significant change at 0.01 significance level in the systolic blood pressure among male subjects of the experimental and control groups; thus Hypothesis 5 has been proved.

HYPOTHESIS 6

The practice of *yoga-nidrā* will decrease the systolic blood pressure in female subjects.

Table 10.6: Systolic BP in Female Subjects

	Mean	sd	"t" Value	Sig. Level
Experimental	109.40	3.44	2.86	At 0.01
Control	116.00	9.77		

Table 10.6 shows the post-mean values as 109.40 of the experimental group and 116 of the control group, and the "t" value is 2.86; a significant change at 0.01 significance level in the systolic blood pressure among female subjects of the experimental and control groups; thus Hypothesis 6 has been proved.

HYPOTHESIS 7

The practice of *yoga-nidrā* will decrease the diastolic blood pressure in male subjects.

Table 10.7: Diastolic BP in Male Subjects

	Mean	sd	"t" Value	Sig. Level
Experimental	75.40	5.68	3.53	At 0.01
Control	78.93	4.20		

Table 10.7 shows the post-mean values as 75.40 of the experimental group and 78.93 of the control group, and the "t" value is 3.53; a significant change at 0.01 significance level in the diastolic blood pressure among male subjects of the experimental and control groups; thus Hypothesis 7 has been proved.

HYPOTHESIS 8

The practice of *yoga-nidrā* will decrease the diastolic blood pressure in female subjects.

Table 10.8: Diastolic BP in Female Subjects

	Mean	sd	"t" Value	Sig. Level
Experimental	72.30	3.13	3.15	At 0.01
Control	76.67	6.17		

Table 10.8 shows the post-mean values as 72.30 of the experimental group and 76.67 of the control group, and the "t" value is 3.15; a significant change at 0.01 significance level in the diastolic blood pressure among female subjects of the experimental and control groups; thus Hypothesis 8 has been proved.

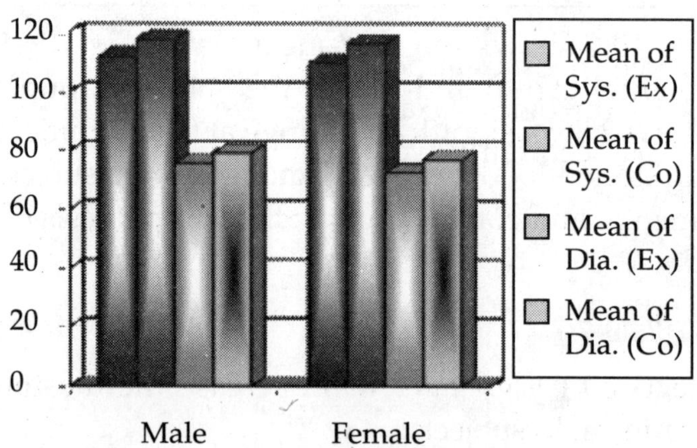

Graph 10.3: Blood Pressure

Graph 10.3 shows the post-values of systolic and diastolic blood pressure of experimental and control group.

Conclusion

The study shows a significant change in the pulse rate, respiration rate, and systolic and diastolic blood-pressure level of the subjects. Through the body–mind relationship, relaxation of body relaxes the entire nervous system. Through the relaxation of central nervous system in *yoga-nidrā,* relaxation in autonomic nervous system takes place, as it reduces the whole physical and mental activities. Reduction in the muscular and neural activities slows down the metabolic rate of the body. During the practice of *yoga-nidrā* due to the relaxed body and mind, muscles become relaxed, arteries of the body become dilated as vasodilatation occurs. Hence the cardiac output as well as cardiac workload reduces; the diastolic and systolic blood pressure with pulse rate comes down as has been seen during the present study. Due to the practice of *yoga-nidrā* relaxed body requires less oxygen accordingly less metabolic activities. Need of the oxygen in the body becomes less; due to that, reduction in the respiration rate has been observed.

Previous researches also support this study as at the Langley Porter Neuropsychiatry Institute in California, Lekh Raj Bali (December 1979) found a reduction in blood pressure levels in hypertensive patients and it continued for twelve months after the *yoga-nidrā* training. Nespor, (August 1981) states that the future role of *yoga-nidrā* in coronary care and management regimes appears to be a major one. The value of the practice of yogic relaxation in prevention of cardiovascular disease has been fairly well recognized and accepted.

11

Alpha EEG, GSR and Yoga-Nidrā

THE EEG measures brainwaves of different frequencies within the brain. Electrodes are placed on specific sites on the scalp to detect and record the electrical impulses within the brain.

A frequency is the number of times a wave repeats itself within a second. It can be compared to the frequencies that you tune into your radio. If any of these frequencies is deficient, excessive or difficult to access, our mental performance can suffer.

Alpha waves are those between 7.5 and 13 Hz. Alpha waves will peak around 10 Hz. Good healthy alpha production promotes mental resourcefulness, aids in the ability to mentally co-ordinate, and enhances overall sense of relaxation and fatigue. In this state one can move quickly and efficiently to accomplish whatever task is at hand. When alpha predominates, most people feel at ease and calm. Alpha appears to bridge the conscious to the subconscious.

It is the major rhythm seen in normal relaxed adults — it is present although the life, especially beyond the thirteenth year when it dominates, the resting tracing.

Alpha rhythms are reported to be derived from the white matter of the brain. The white matter can be considered as part of the brain that connects all parts with each other.

Alpha is a common state for the brain and occurs whenever a person is alert (it is a marker for alertness and sleep), but not actively processing information. Alpha rhythms are the strongest over the occipital (back of the head) cortex and also over frontal cortex.

Alpha has been linked to extroversion (introverts show less), creativity (creative subjects show alpha when listening and coming to a solution for creative problems), and mental work.

When our alpha is within normal ranges we tend to also experience good moods, see the world truthfully and have a sense of calmness. Alpha is one of the brain's most important frequencies to learn and use information taught in the classroom and on the job. One can increase alpha by closing your eyes or deep breathing or decrease alpha by thinking or calculating.

In this scenario, alpha would represent neutral or idle. Alpha allows us to shift easily from one task to another.

Galvanic Skin Response (GSR): a change in the electrical properties of the skin in response to stress or anxiety can be measured either by recording the electrical resistance of the skin or by recording weak currents generated by the body. It can also be understood as a drop in the electrical resistance of the skin, widely used as an index of autonomic reaction.

Again, stratified-quota sampling was used in this study. The total sample covered for the purpose of the present study belonged to the students of PG Yoga classes from Dev Sanskriti Vishwavidyalaya, Shantikunj, Haridwar; who were of between 20-30 age group and 110 in numbers (fifty-five males and fifty-five females). They were further divided into forty males and forty females in experimental group; as well as fifteen males and fifteen females in control group.

In the study, control-group research design was adopted. To measure the alpha EEG, alpha EEG biofeedback was used, which is a process of monitoring and displaying to an individual the ongoing alpha EEG activity generated by his brain. Its most common clinical application is to redress a chronic mental posture constituting a component of psychosomatic or psychological disorder. Many individuals suffering from stress-related disorders exhibit excessive mental arousal and rumination associated with an inappropriate degree of desynchronized high frequency (beta) activity. The EEG potentials emitted by the human brain provide one of the activities of human central nervous system.

In alpha EEG feedback, EEG activity is detected by surface electrodes attached to the scalp, and then amplified, analysed and translated into visual and auditory feedback displays. By receiving immediate and continuous information reflecting alpha EEG frequency and amplitude fluctuations, an individual can learn to recognize physiological states.

To measure the GSR of the subjects, GSR biofeedback has been brought in application, which is utilized clinically as a convenient indicator of emotional responses and as a training tool for generalized reduction of sympathetic activity and the treatment of related psychosomatic and psychological disorders. It can play a major role in improving the patient's awareness of both the objective physiological indications of inappropriate stress responses and the mechanisms involved in their generation and maintenance.

Hypothesis and Result

HYPOTHESIS 9

The practice of *yoga-nidrā* will positively increase alpha EEG of the male subjects.

Table 11.1: Alpha EEG in Male Subjects

	Mean	sd	"t" Value	Sig. Level
Experimental	9.54	4.97	7.2	At 0.01
Control	5.55	2.40		

Table 11.1 shows the post-mean values as 9.54 of the experimental group and 5.55 of the control group, and the "t" value is 7.2; a significant change at 0.01 significance level in the Alpha EEG of the male subjects of the experimental and control groups; thus Hypothesis 9 has been proved.

HYPOTHESIS 10

The practice of *yoga-nidrā* will positively increase alpha EEG of the female subjects.

Table 11.2: Alpha EEG for Female Subjects

	Mean	sd	"t" Value	Sig. Level
Experimental	8.97	3.66	2.2	At 0.01
Control	6.35	2.19		

Table 11.2 shows the post-mean values as 8.97 of the experimental group and 6.35 of the control group, and the "t" value is 2.2; a significant change at 0.01 significance level in the alpha EEG of the female subjects of the experimental and control groups; thus Hypothesis 10 has been proved.

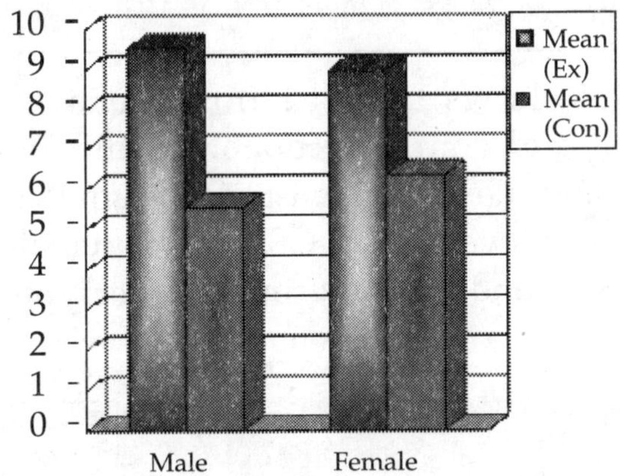

Graph 11.1: Alpha EEG

Graph 11.1 shows the post-mean values of the alpha EEG of the experimental and control groups.

HYPOTHESIS 11

The practice of *yoga-nidrā* will positively increase the level of GSR in the male subjects.

Table 11.3: GSR in Male Subjects

	Mean	sd	"t" Value	Sig. Level
Experimental	187.68	161.69	4.58	At 0.01
Control	85.53	42.04		

Table 11.3 shows that the post-mean values of the experimental and control groups are 187.68 and 85.53, respectively, and the "t" value is 4.58; a significant change at

0.01 significance level in the GSR of the male subjects of the experimental and control groups; thus Hypothesis 11 has been proved.

HYPOTHESIS 12

The practice of *yoga-nidrā* will positively increase the level of GSR in the female subjects.

Table 11.4: GSR Level in Female Subjects

	Mean	sd	"t" Value	Sig. Level
Experimental	485.53	868.50	3.44	At 0.01
Control	178.43	136.95		

Table 11.4 shows that the post-mean values of the experimental and control groups are 485.53 and 178.43, respectively, and the "t" value is 3.44; a significant change at 0.01 significance level in the GSR of the female subjects of the experimental and control groups; thus Hypothesis 12 has been proved.

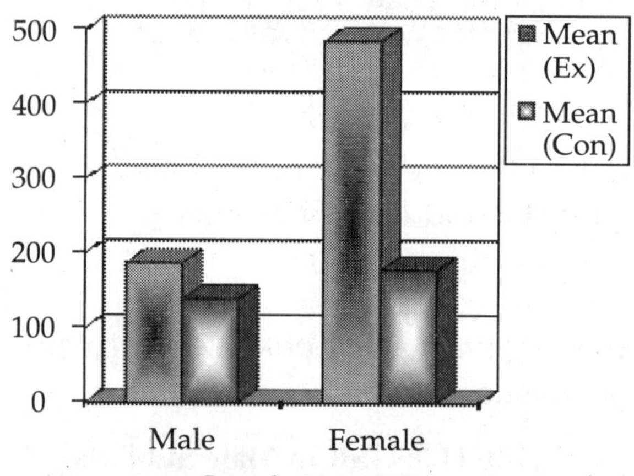

Graph 11.2: GSR

Graph 11.2 shows the post-mean values of the GSR of the experimental and control groups.

Conclusion

The study also shows a significant change in the alpha EEG level of the subjects. EEG measures minute electrical activity in the brain in the form of waves. The frequency of brain-activity waves has been shown to alter according to the state of consciousness and state of mind the subject is in. Beta activity is normally noted in the awake working state. With physical relaxation beta activity is taken up by alpha activity, and as the person goes into different stages of sleep the activity changes to theta and also may exhibit delta activity in deep sleep. Sannyasi Mangalteertham (1998) concluded on the basis of his study that the practice of *yoga-nidrā* brings alpha dominance in the brain, which is characterized by mental relaxation.

As we know the practice of *yoga-nidrā* is the intermediate stage of awakened and sleep, and it is the stage of the brain when it produces alpha waves. As Roney-Dougal (2011) observed in a study, initial EEG showed beta activity prominently with intermittent alpha activity. With the advancement of *yoga-nidrā,* beta activity was slowly replaced by alpha activity and still further by smooth well-formed alpha activity. After thirty sessions of *yoga-nidrā,* gain of alpha activity was better and with further advancement of *yoga-nidrā* intermittent theta activity was noted intermixed with alpha activity, suggestive of deep state of relaxation.

A significant change also showed in this study is in the GSR level of the subjects. As we know GSR is a change in the electrical properties of the skin in response to stress or anxiety; and it can be measured either by recording the electrical resistance of the skin or by recording weak currents generated by the body. It can also be understood as a drop in the electrical resistance of the skin, widely used as an index of autonomic reaction. Jennifer Macey (2005) has made a direct connection between the nervous and immune system. The study reported that stress leads to a build up of a hormone that inhibits the body's ability to fight off bacteria and viruses. Since practice of *yoga-nidrā* is able to reduce the stress and anxiety of the practitioners, and because of its total relaxation effect on the physical and mental state, it improves the GSR of the subjects.

12

Haematological Profile and Yoga-Nidrā

HAEMATOLOGICAL information assesses the body's ability to carry oxygen, provide immunological surveillance and prevent haemorrhage. Typical tests include complete blood counts, which measure the number of red blood cells or haemoglobin, white blood cells or Total Leucocytes Counts (TLC) and platelets.

Haemoglobin is a red pigment in red blood cells that can bind with oxygen and is largely responsible for the blood's oxygen-carrying capacity. Haemoglobin is composed of four polypeptide, two alpha (α) and two beta (β) chains.

It is the iron-containing pigment in red blood cells that carries oxygen to the tissue cells. A reduction in red blood cells decreases haemoglobin. A decreased haemoglobin concentration is called anemia. The decrease in haemoglobin concentration reduces the oxygen-carrying capacity of blood. If severe, this decreased capacity may limit a person's capacity to exert them. Normal values of blood haemoglobin are 13-18 gm per 100 ml of blood in men. Women, on an average, have almost 10 per cent less haemoglobin than men.

Erythrocyte Sedimentation Rate (ESR) is a measurement of how quickly red blood cells fall to the bottom of a test tube. When swelling and inflammation are present, the blood's proteins clump together and become heavier than normal. Thus, when measured, they fall and settle faster at the bottom of the test tube. Generally, the faster the blood cells fall, the more severe the inflammation. The distance red blood cells travel in one hour in a sample of blood as they settle to the bottom of a test tube. It is also called sedimentation rate. The sedimentation rate is increased in inflammation, infection, cancer, rheumatic diseases, and diseases of the blood and bone marrow.

TLC means total leucocytes counts. Leucocytes are the white blood cells, which are transparent and not coloured. It fights against the infections. There are 6,000-10,000 (with an average of 8,000) leucocytes in each cubic millimetre of blood. DLC is differential leucocytes counts. Leucocytes or white blood cells are neutrophils or polymorphs, basophils, lymphocytes and monocytes. The numbers of blood cells in each cubic millimetre of blood are as follows:

Leukocytes	Per cent	Average (%)
Granulocytes		
Neutrophil or polymorph	60-70	66
Eosinophil cells	1-4	3
Basophil cell	0-2	1
Non-Granulocytes		
Lymphocytes	20-30	25
Monocytes	4-8	5

Stratified-quota sampling was used in this study. The total sample covered for the purpose of the present study belonged to the students of PG Yoga classes from Dev Sanskriti Vishwavidyalaya, Shantikunj, Haridwar; who were of between 20-30 age group and 110 in numbers (fifty-five males and fifty-five females). They were further divided into forty males and forty females in experimental group; as well as fifteen males and fifteen females in control group.

In the study, control-group research design was used. To measure the haemoglobin, haemometer (Sahili Method); for ESR, Westergren Tube; and for TLC and DLC, monocular/binocular microscope were used.

Hypothesis and Result

HYPOTHESIS 13

The practice of *yoga-nidrā* will positively increase the level of haemoglobin in male subjects.

Table 12.1: Haemoglobin Level in Male Subjects

	Mean	sd	"t" Value	Sig. Level
Experimental	13.60	0.65	3.22	At 0.01
Control	12.87	0.74		

Table 12.1 shows that the post-mean values of the experimental and control groups are 13.6 and 12.87, respectively, and the "t" value is 3.22; a significant change at 0.01 significance level in the haemoglobin among male subjects of the experimental and control groups; thus Hypothesis 13 has been proved.

HYPOTHESIS 14

The practice of *yoga-nidrā* will positively increase the level of haemoglobin in female subjects.

Table 12.2: Haemoglobin Level in Female Subjects

	Mean	sd	"t" Value	Sig. Level
Experimental	12.69	0.74	2.51	At 0.01
Control	11.77	0.90		

Table 12.2 shows that the post-mean values of the experimental and control groups are 12.69 and 11.77, respectively, and the "t" value is 2.51; a significant change at 0.01 significance level in the haemoglobin among female subjects of the experimental and control groups; thus Hypothesis 14 has been proved.

Graph 12.1 shows the post-values of haemoglobin of the experimental and control groups.

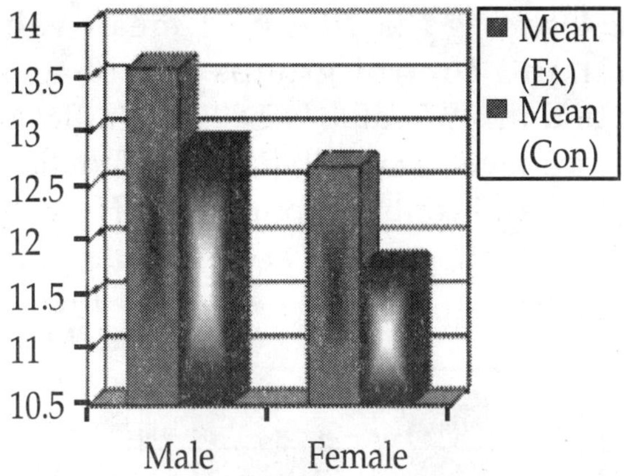

Graph 12.1: Haemoglobin

HYPOTHESIS 15

There is a significant relationship between the practice of *yoga-nidrā* and ESR in male subjects.

Table 12.3: ESR Level in Male Subjects

	Mean	sd	"t" Value	Sig. Level
Experimental	2.87	1.81	5.06	At 0.01
Control	11.43	12.58		

Table 12.3 shows that the post-mean values of the experimental and control groups are 2.87 and 11.43, respectively, and the "t" value is 5.06; a significant change at 0.01 significance level in the ESR of the male subjects of the experimental and control groups; thus Hypothesis 15 has been proved.

HYPOTHESIS 16

There is a significant relationship between the practice of *yoga-nidrā* and ESR in female subjects.

Table 12.4: ESR Level in Female Subjects

	Mean	sd	"t" Value	Sig. Level
Experimental	10.40	11.10	2.82	At 0.01
Control	12.15	13.95		

Table 12.4 shows that the post-mean values of the experimental and control groups are 10.40 and 12.15, respectively, and the "t" value is 2.82; a significant change at 0.01 significance level in the ESR of the female subjects of the experimental and control groups; thus Hypothesis 16 has been proved.

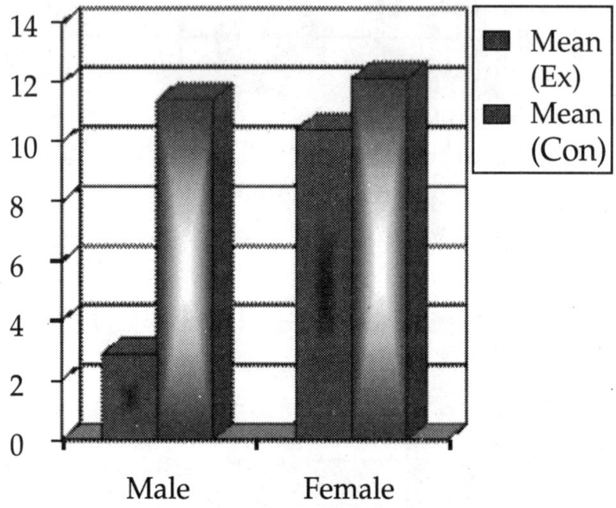

Graph 12.2: ESR

Graph 12.2 shows the post-values of ESR of the experimental and control groups.

HYPOTHESIS 17

There is a significant relationship between the practice of *yoga-nidrā* and TLC in male subjects.

Table 12.5: TLC Level in Male Subjects

	Mean	sd	"t" Value	Sig level
Experimental	7770.00	980.37	5.01	At 0.01
Control	6786.67	843.35		

Table 12.5 shows that the post-mean values of the experimental and control groups are 7770 and 6786.67, respectively, and the "t" value is 5.01; there is a significant change at 0.01 significance level in the TLC of the male subjects of the experimental and control groups; thus Hypothesis 17 has been proved.

HYPOTHESIS 18

There is a significant relationship between the practice of *yoga-nidrā* and TLC in female subjects.

Table 12.6: TLC Level in Female Subjects

	Mean	sd	"t" Value	Sig. Level
Experimental	7470.00	532.22	1.67	At 0.01
Control	6786.667	1604.40		

Table 12.6 shows that the post-mean values of the experimental and control groups are 7470 and 6786.67, respectively, and the "t" value is 1.67; there is a significant change at 0.01 significance level in the TLC of the female subjects of the experimental and control groups; thus Hypothesis 18 has been proved.

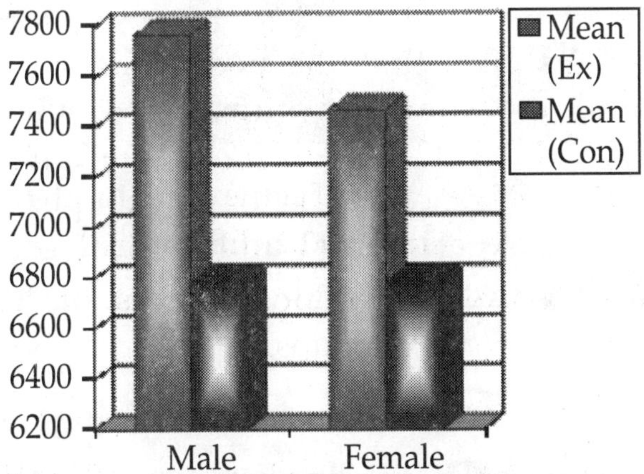

Graph 12.3: TLC

Graph 12.3 shows the post-mean values of TLC of the experimental and control groups.

HYPOTHESIS 19

There is a significant relationship between the practice of *yoga-nidrā* and DLC (polymorph) in male subjects.

Table 12.7: DLC (Polymorph) Level in Male Subjects

	Mean	sd	"t" Value	Sig. Level
Experimental	64.10	5.49	0.47	At 0.01
Control	63.07	4.98		

Table 12.7 shows that the post-mean values of the experimental and control groups are 64.1 and 63.07, respectively, and the "t" value is 0.47; there is no significant change at 0.01 significance level in the polymorph of the male subjects of the experimental and control groups; thus Hypothesis 19 has been rejected.

HYPOTHESIS 20

There is a significant relationship between the practice of *yoga-nidrā* and DLC in female subjects.

Table 12.8: DLC (Polymorph) Level in Female Subjects

	Mean	sd	"t" Value	Sig. Level
Experimental	63.48	4.53	0.26	At 0.01
Control	62.87	10.32		

Table 12.8 shows that the post-mean values of the experimental and control groups are 63.48 and 62.87, respectively, and the "t" value is 0.26; there is no significant change at 0.01 significance level in the polymorph of the female subjects of the experimental and control groups; thus Hypothesis 20 has been rejected.

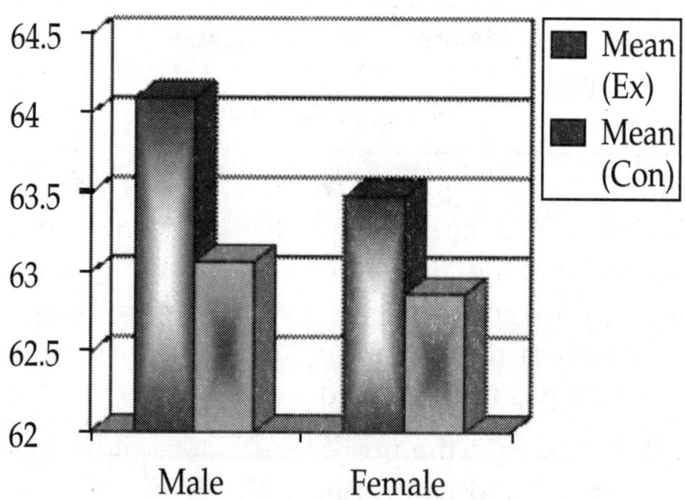

Graph 12.4: DLC (polymorph)

Graph 12.4 shows the post-mean values of polymorphs of experimental and control group.

HYPOTHESIS 21

There is a significant relationship between the practice of *yoga-nidrā* and DLC (Lymphocyte) in male subjects.

Table 12.9: DLC (Lymphocyte) Level in Male Subjects

	Mean	sd	"t" Value	Sig. Level
Experimental	33.45	5.21	1.28	At 0.01
Control	32.60	5.87		

Table 12.9 shows that the post-mean values of the experimental and control groups are 33.45 and 32.60, respectively, and the "t" value is 1.28; there is a significant change at 0.01 significance level in the lymphocyte of the male subjects of the experimental and control groups; thus Hypothesis 21 has been proved.

HYPOTHESIS 22

There is a significant relationship between the practice of *yoga-nidrā* and DLC in female subjects.

Table 12.10: DLC (Lymphocyte) Level in Female Subjects

	Mean	sd	"t" Value	Sig. Level
Experimental	33.78	5.20	3.19	At 0.01
Control	36.27	3.71		

Table 12.10 shows that the post-mean values of the experimental and control groups are 33.78 and 36.27, respectively, and the "t" value is 3.19; there is a significant change at 0.01 significance level in the lymphocyte of the female subjects of the experimental and control groups; thus Hypothesis 22 has been proved.

Graph 12.5 shows the post-mean values of lymphocyte of the experimental and control groups.

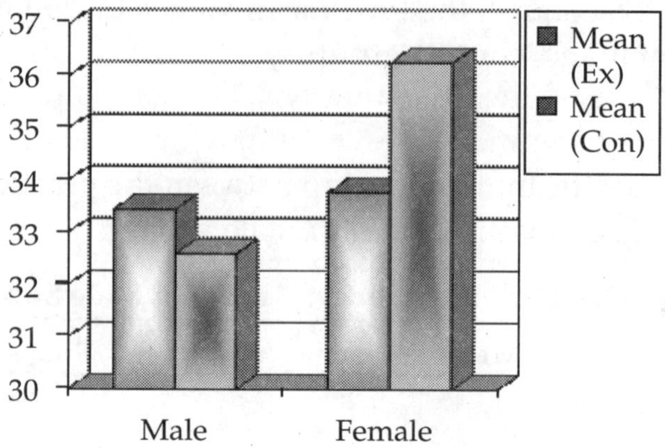

Graph 12.5: DLC (lymphocyte)

HYPOTHESIS 23

There is a significant relationship between the practice of *yoga-nidrā* and DLC (monocyte) in male subjects.

Table 12.11: DLC (Monocyte) Level in Male Subjects

	Mean	sd	"t" Value	Sig. Level
Experimental	4.63	1.43	2.14	At 0.01
Control	5.53	1.51		

Table 12.11 shows that the post-mean values of the experimental and control groups are 4.63 and 5.53, respectively, and the "t" value is 2.14; there is no significant change at 0.01 significance level in the monocyte of the male subjects of the experimental and control groups; thus Hypothesis 23 has been rejected.

HYPOTHESIS 24

There is a significant relationship between the practice of *yoga-nidrā* and DLC in female subjects.

Table 12.12: DLC (Monocyte) Level in Female Subjects

	Mean	sd	"t" Value	Sig. Level
Experimental	4.28	1.75	3.95	At 0.01
Control	5.07	1.03		

Table 12.12 shows that the post-mean values of the experimental and control groups are 4.28 and 5.07, respectively, and the "t" value is 3.95; there is no significant change at 0.01 significance level in the monocyte of the female subjects of the experimental and control groups; thus Hypothesis 24 has been rejected.

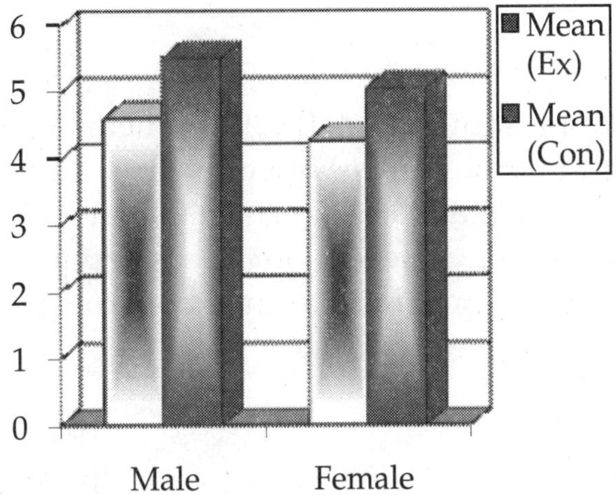

Graph 12.6: DLC (monocyte)

Graph 12.6 shows the post-mean values of monocytes of the experimental and control groups.

HYPOTHESIS 25

There is a significant relationship between the practice of *yoga-nidrā* and DLC (eosinophil) in male subjects.

Table 12.13: DLC (Eosinophil) Level in Male Subjects

	Mean	sd	"t" Value	Sig. Level
Experimental	2.0	1.01	2.68	At 0.01
Control	1.47	0.64		

Table 12.13 shows that the post-mean values of the experimental and control groups are 2.00 and 1.47, respectively, and the "t" value is 2.68; there is a significant change at 0.01 significance level in the eosinophil of the male subjects of the experimental and control groups; thus Hypothesis 25 has been proved.

HYPOTHESIS 26

There is a significant relationship between the practice of *yoga-nidrā* and DLC (eosinophil) in female subjects.

Table 12.14: DLC (Eosinophil) Level in Female Subjects

	Mean	sd	"t" Value	Sig. Level
Experimental	2.05	1.93	2.89	At 0.01
Control	1.53	0.99		

Table 12.14 shows that the post-mean values of the experimental and control groups are 2.05 and 1.53, respectively, and the "t" value is 2.89; there is a significant change at 0.01 significance level in the eosinophil of the female subjects of the experimental and control groups; thus Hypothesis 26 has been proved.

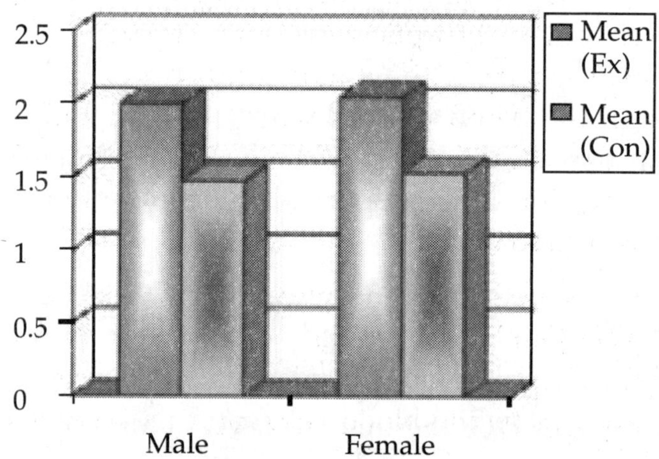

Graph 12.7: DLC (eosinophil)

Graph 12.7 shows the post-mean values of eosinophil of the experimental and control groups.

Conclusion

The study shows a significant change in the haemoglobin level of the subjects. As haemoglobin is a protein-based component of red blood cells, it is primarily responsible for transferring oxygen from the lungs to the rest of the body. Haemoglobin is actually the reason for red blood cells appear red, although oxygen-rich blood is noticeably brighter than the depleted blood returning to the heart and lungs. Fresh haemoglobin is produced in the bone marrow as needed, based on our food intake. Here *yoga-nidrā* does not directly affect the haemoglobin level of the subjects. It is a well-known scientific fact that insufficient oxygen in the body can bring several changes like erythropoietin is secreted by kidney and increases production of red blood cells in the bone marrow. Practice of *yoga-nidrā* reduces the respiration rate due to the relaxed muscular and metabolic activities. This is the region which results in significant change in haemoglobin of the subjects

Hence practice of *yoga-nidrā* not only relaxes the body, mind and emotions; it relaxes the consciousness also. Through the holistic relaxation of all the internal organs, it improves the digestion as well as absorption and assimilation of food. When iron is absorbed from the small intestine, it immediately combines in the blood plasma with a beta globulin; which shows an increased number of haemoglobin as a result of proper absorption. The proper food consumption is one of the reasons behind it.

The study shows a significant change in the TLC and ESR of the subjects. Our bodies have a special system for combating the different infectious and toxic agents. This is comprised of blood leukocytes (white blood cells) and tissue cells derived from leukocytes.

When tensions, conflicts and frustrations of the mind manifest in the form of physical symptoms, those diseases are termed as psychosomatic diseases. *Yoga-nidrā* aims at releasing the suppressed and repressed conflicts from the unconscious, thereby relaxing the mind. When the potent cause (tense mind) of psychosomatic disorders is managed, the disease can also be cured. The practice of various stages of *yoga-nidrā,* like *saṅkalpa,* muscular relaxation, breath awareness and guided imagery has been found to be a significant and effective mode of therapy. As *yoga-nidrā* is a complete relaxation process of the body and mind, it increases the immunity of a person, hence the change in the ESR and TLC should be positive; which has been found in this study. The following studies support our study.

Jennifer Macey (2005) has made a direct connection between the nervous and immune system. Her study reported that stress leads to a build up of a hormone that inhibits the body's ability to fight off bacteria and viruses. Erythrocyte sedimentation rate decreases and increase in total leukocyte count is the result of a strong immunity which comes by stress release of physical, mental and emotional states.

Erskine Milliss and Schonell (1981) and Gupta et al. (1979) reported that eighteen out of twenty-seven asthmatic patients showed improvement in respiratory function and greater freedom of breathing after intensive training in *yoga-nidrā*, and 63 per cent had definite relaxation and dilation of the bronchial tubes when tested on a spirometer. Jansson (1979) reported that after three weeks of relaxation training the symptoms of colonic irritability significantly reduced. In the case of cardiac patients, Cooper and Aygen (1979) reported that *yoga-nidrā* significantly lowered levels of serum cholesterol in cardiac patients. Researches also show that the practice of *yoga-nidrā* lowers the elevated blood pressure levels of hypertensive patients (Datey et al. (1977) and Bali (1979)). In this way, the practice of *yoga-nidrā* effectively manages various psychosomatic diseases.

No significant change was seen in the DLC (polymorphs) and DLC (monocytes). However, there is a significant change in lymphocytes and eosinophils. Though there is a change in polymorphs and monocytes it is not significant because the pre-value of these parameters has not changed much from the ideal number of the blood cell counts. The change is only in lymphocytes and eosinophils because the practice of *yoga-nidrā* brings the system mechanism towards normal due to proper metabolism and proper nervous supply.

13

Yoga-Nidrā for Memory and Well-being

GENERAL well-being may be defined as a subjective feeling of contentment, happiness, satisfaction with life's experiences and of one's role in the world of work, sense of achievement, utility, belongingness, and no distress, dissatisfaction or worry, etc. These things are difficult to evaluate objectively. It may be well maintained in adverse circumstances and conversely, may be lost in favourable situations. It is related to but not dependent upon the physical/physiological conditions.

Memory is a property of the human mind: the ability to retain information. Memory is much studied in cognitive psychology and neuroscience. There are multiple classifications for memory based on duration, nature and retrieval of perceived items.

Memory is defined as: "The ability, process, or act of remembering or recalling; especially the ability to reproduce what has been learned or explained," — *American Psychiatric Glossary*, p. 126. The question — "What is a memory?" — had become increasingly controversial in the last decade. As Post Traumatic Stress Disorder (PTSD) and dissociative disorder clients report delayed and dissociated memories of childhood trauma, the accuracy or validity of these memories has been questioned. At present, there is no reliable scientific method to assess the self-report of traumatic events. While the presence of corroborating evidence (or witnesses) may support a survivor's memories, it does not in itself determine.

Short-term memory, sometimes referred to as "primary" or "active" memory, is that part of memory which stores a limited amount of information for a limited amount of time (roughly 30-45 seconds). This can be contrasted to long-term memory, in which a seemingly unlimited amount of information is stored indefinitely. It can be described as the capacity (or capacities) for holding in mind, in an active, highly available state, a small amount of information.

As we did previously, the stratified-quota sampling method was used in this study also. The total sample covered for the purpose of the present study belonged to the students of PG Yoga classes from Dev Sanskriti Vishwavidyalaya, Shantikunj, Haridwar; who were of between 20-30 age group and 110 in numbers (fifty-five males and fifty-five females). They were further divided into forty males and forty females in experimental group; as well as fifteen males and fifteen females in control group.

In the study, control-group research design was adopted. To measure the general well-being, PGI General Well Being Measure (standard questionnaire), developed by Santosh K. Verma and Amita Verma, Chandigarh, was used.

To measure the immediate memory, C.M. Bhatia's Performance Test of Intelligence was applied.

Hypothesis and Result

HYPOTHESIS 27

The practice of *yoga-nidrā* will positively affect the general well-being of the male subjects.

Table 13.1: General Well-being Level of Male Subjects

	Mean	sd	"t" Value	Sig. Level
Experimental	16.08	2.97	1.98	At 0.01
Control	14.33	4.20		

Table 13.1 shows that the post-mean values of the experimental and control groups are 16.08 and 14.33, respectively, and the "t" value is 1.98; there is a significant change at 0.01 significance level in the general well-being of the male subjects of the experimental and control groups; thus Hypothesis 27 has been proved.

HYPOTHESIS 28

The practice of *yoga-nidrā* will positively affect the general well-being of the female subjects.

Table 13.2: General Well-being Level of Female Subjects

	Mean	sd	"t" Value	Sig. Level
Experimental	16.15	2.18	4.15	At 0.01
Control	10.67	5.96		

Table 13.2 shows that the post-mean values of the experimental and control groups are 16.15 and 10.67, respectively, and the "t" value is 4.15; there is a significant change at 0.01 significance level in the general well-being of the female subjects of the experimental and control groups; thus Hypothesis 28 has been proved.

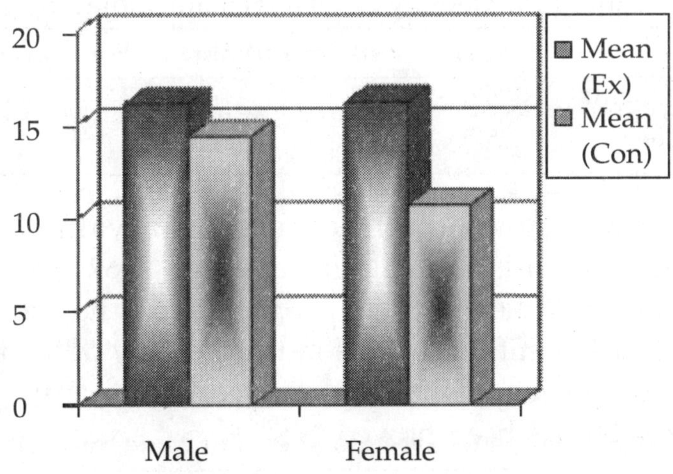

Graph 13.1: General well-being Level

Graph 13.1 shows the post-mean values of general well-being of the experimental and control groups.

HYPOTHESIS 29

The practice of *yoga-nidrā* will positively affect the memory of the male subjects.

Table 13.3: Memory Level of Male Subjects

	Mean	sd	"t" Value	Sig. Level
Experimental	6.59	0.88	8.42	At 0.01
Control	5.13	0.92		

Table 13.3 shows that the post-mean values of the experimental and control groups are 6.59 and 5.13, respectively, and the "t" value is 8.42; there is a significant change at 0.01 significance level in the memory of the male subjects of the experimental and control groups; thus Hypothesis 29 has been proved.

HYPOTHESIS 30

The practice of *yoga-nidrā* will positively affect the memory of the female subjects.

Table 13.4: Memory Level of Female Subjects

	Mean	sd	"t" Value	Sig. Level
Experimental	6.62	1.07	6.45	At 0.0
Control	5.53	1.18		

Table 13.4 shows that the post-mean values of the experimental and control groups are 6.62 and 5.53, respectively, and the "t" value is 6.45; there is no significant change at 0.01 significance level in the memory of the female subjects of the experimental and control groups; thus Hypothesis 30 has been proved.

Graph 13.2 shows the post-mean values of memory of the experimental and control groups.

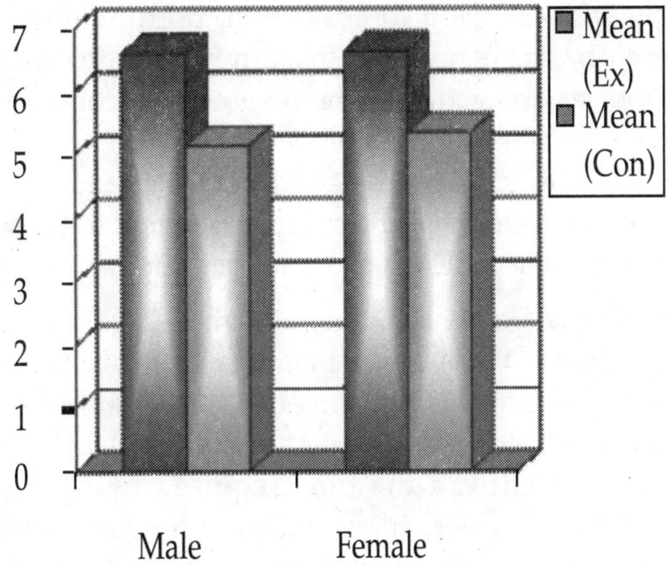

Graph 13.2: Memory

Conclusion

A significant change has been observed in the general well-being level of the subjects during this study. General well-being may be defined as the subjective feeling of contentment, happiness, satisfaction with life's experiences and of one's role in the world of work, sense of achievement, utility, belongingness, no distress, dissatisfaction or worry, etc.

A high percentage of people remains in a state of tension and frustration. This continuous level of tension in the body, mind and emotions predisposes the individual towards psychological and psychosomatic disorders. Practice of *yoga-nidrā* releases all the worries and tensions, and enhances the contentment and the sense of happiness. This is the reason behind the positive change in the general well-being of the subjects.

There is a significant change in the memory of the subjects. The technique of *yoga-nidrā* is helpful in increasing the learning capacity and memory power. Here the original memory may not be changed but attention and awareness towards learning improve through the relaxation of mind and consciousness.

When *yoga-nidrā* is used in education, both hemispheres of the student's brain are involved in learning the subject, whereas in classroom teaching the left hemisphere functions more. In this way, the practice of *yoga-nidrā* involves the total mind in learning. The thoughtlessness condition of the mind, during the practice, brings in a significant improvement in the memory of the subjects. The following researches support our study.

Veena Verma (Sannyasi Soumya Shakti) (2004) states on the basis of a study that *yoga-nidrā* has a positive impact in enhancing the memory. Ostrander and Schroeder (1973) said that, "using the technique of *yoga-nidrā* it was possible to teach a foreign language in one-fifth of the time required by conventional methods". Schoolteachers in several countries are using *yoga-nidrā* to augment the capacities of receptivity and attention, and to awaken the joy of learning in their young students. Flak (1978) reported that techniques such as rotation of awareness and visualization heighten the capacity for relaxation and interest among schoolchildren. This method may be good for the intelligent students. The technique of *yoga-nidrā* can be used as an educational tool for the children, where the knowledge is transmitted directly into the subconscious mind.

14

Stress–Anxiety and Yoga-Nidrā

STRESS (roughly the opposite of relaxation) is a medical term for a wide range of strong external stimuli, both physiological and psychological, which can cause a physiological response called a general adaptation syndrome, first described in 1936 by Hans Seley in the journal, *Nature*.

An emotionally disruptive or upsetting condition occurring in response to adverse external influences and capable of affecting physical health which can be characterized by increased heart rate, a rise in blood pressure, muscular tension, irritability and depression.

Anxiety is a complex combination of the feeling of fear, apprehension and worry, often accompanied by physical sensations such as palpitations, chest pain and/or shortness of breath. It may exist as a primary disorder or may be associated with other medical problems including other psychiatric disorders.

Anxiety is a feeling of apprehension, worry, uneasiness or dread. Excess anxiety interferes with a child's ability to function normally. This is common in children who have been abused and neglected. Treatment can include medication and/or therapy. Almost all recently placed adoptive children will have some degree of anxiety, so will the parents.

Stratified-quota sampling was used in this study. The total sample covered for the purpose of the present study belonged to the students of PG Yoga classes from Dev Sanskriti Vishwavidyalaya, Shantikunj, Haridwar; who were of 20-30 age group and 110 in numbers (fifty-five males and fifty-five females). They were further divided into forty males and forty females in experimental group; as well as fifteen males and fifteen females in control group.

In the study, control-group research design was adopted.

To measure the test psychological parameters — anxiety and stress — we have applied the Eight State Questionnaire, developed by Barton, Cattell and Curran in 1973 and adopted by S.D. Kapoor (published and reprinted in India by The Psycho Centre, New Delhi).

Hypothesis and Result

HYPOTHESIS 31

The practice of *yoga-nidrā* will decrease the anxiety level of the male subjects.

Table 14.1: Anxiety Level of Male Subjects

	Mean	sd	"t" Value	Sig. Level
Experimental	4.90	1.22	2.5	At 0.01
Control	5.60	1.45		

Table 14.1 shows that the post-mean values of the experimental and control groups are 4.9 and 5.6, respectively, and the "t" value is 2.5; there is a significant change at 0.01 significance level in the anxiety of the male subjects of the experimental and control groups; thus Hypothesis 31 has been proved.

HYPOTHESIS 32

The practice of *yoga-nidrā* will decrease the anxiety of the female subjects.

Table 14.2: Anxiety Level of Female Subjects

	Mean	sd	"t" Value	Sig. Level
Experimental	4.87	1.13	2.2	At 0.01
Control	5.28	1.41		

Table 14.2 shows that the post-mean values of the experimental and control groups are 4.87 and 5.28, respectively, and the "t" value is 2.2; there is a significant change at 0.01 significance level in the anxiety of the female subjects of the experimental and control groups; thus Hypothesis 32 has been proved.

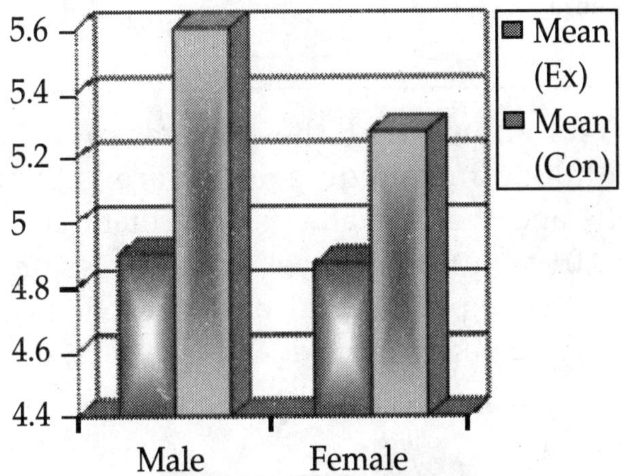

Graph 14.1: Anxiety

Graph 14.1 shows the post-mean values of anxiety of the experimental and control groups.

HYPOTHESIS 33

The practice of *yoga-nidrā* will decrease the stress of the male subjects.

Table 14.3: Stress Level of Male Subjects

	Mean	sd	"t" Value	Sig. Level
Experimental	4.63	1.43	2.14	At 0.01
Control	5.53	1.51		

Table 14.3 shows that the post-mean values of the experimental and control groups are 4.63 and 5.53, respectively, and the "t" value is 2.14; there is a significant change at 0.01 significance level in the stress of the male subjects of the experimental and control groups; thus Hypothesis 33 has been proved.

HYPOTHESIS 34

The practice of *yoga-nidrā* will decrease the stress of the female subjects.

Table 14.4: Stress Level of Female Subjects

	Mean	sd	"t" Value	Sig. Level
Experimental	4.28	1.75	3.95	At 0.01
Control	5.28	1.41		

Table 14.4 shows that the post-mean values of the experimental and control groups are 4.28 and 5.28, respectively, and the "t" value is 3.95; there is a significant change at 0.01 significance level in the stress of the female subjects of the experimental and control groups; thus Hypothesis 34 has been proved.

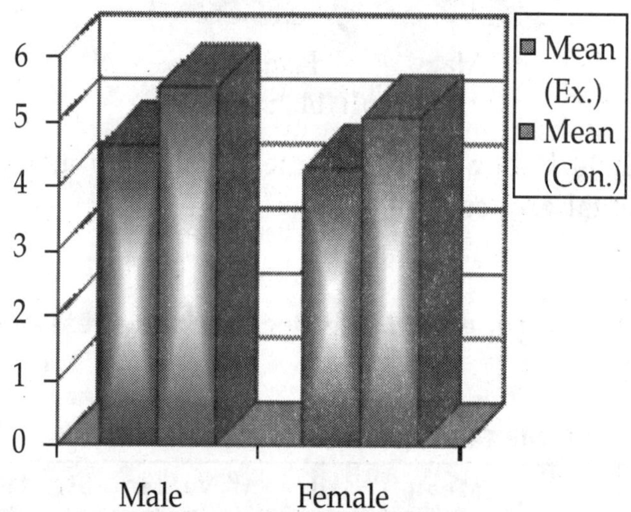

Graph 14.2: Stress

Graph 14.2 shows the post-mean values of stress of the experimental and control groups.

Conclusion

A significant change has been observed in the anxiety and stress levels of the subjects during this study. As we know anxiety is a complex combination of the feeling of fear, apprehension and worry often accompanied by physical sensations such as palpitations, chest pain and/or shortness of breath. It may exist as a primary disorder or may be associated with other medical problems including other psychiatric disorders.

Anxiety is a feeling of apprehension, worry, uneasiness or dread. Stress is a cognitive or emotional response made by the individual towards any situation, which demands adjustment. As the demands of the situation exceed the ability of the individual, distress results, which may manifest in mental and physical symptoms of abnormality. The practice of *yoga-nidrā* helps in building up the coping ability. Hence it is a practice of total relaxation; it stops all unnecessary thinking process, which is the main factor behind all psychological imbalances. The practitioner of *yoga-nidrā* slowly becomes aware of the inherent dormant potentialities and thus prevents himself from becoming a victim of distress.

During stress, the sympathetic nervous system becomes activated due to which the organism adopts the "fight or flight" mechanism. In normal circumstances, the parasympathetic system takes over after the emergency goes. But mostly it has been seen that the sympathetic system remains active most of the time resulting in the experience of distress (Shelley 1974). The following researches support our findings.

Udupa (1977) suggests that stress-related disorders evolve gradually through four stages. In the first stage, psychological symptoms like anxiety and irritability arise due to over activation of the sympathetic nervous system. The second stage is characterized by related physical symptoms like high blood pressure and increased heart rate. In the third stage, the abnormalities manifest clinically in the organ systems. In the last stage, severe symptoms in particular organs appear which need long-term medical management.

Bahrke (1979) also concluded on the basis of his study that the practice of yogic relaxation has been found to effectively reduce tension and improve the psychological well-being of sufferers from anxiety.

Swami Satyananda Saraswati (1998) has said that *yoga-nidrā* is now prescribed by doctors in many countries both as a preventive and curative therapy in the first three stages of stress-related diseases.

In *yoga-nidrā* an attempt is made to activate the parasympathetic system, and slowly a balance between the sympathetic and parasympathetic systems is achieved by inducing complete physical, emotional and mental relaxation. In this way, the practice of *yoga-nidrā* counteracts stress. Carrington et al. (1980) concluded that *yoga-nidrā* has its most widespread application as a preventive measure to be practised by healthy, active people as a means of relieving accumulated tensions, increasing stress resistance and overall efficiency, and preventing the development of stress-related diseases.

15

Psychological Changes and Yoga-Nidrā

MENTAL faculties are the most precious bequests of the Almighty bestowed upon us. However, the belief that we can't expand or elevate the god-gifted mental potentials we are born with is not correct. The difference in people's intellectual and other mental abilities is only that of the degree of arousal and activation of the grand powers indwelling in the human self. This difference is not due to the structure of the brain, inheritance or destiny. Rather, it is a reflection of the extent of dormancy or activation of its unlimited potentials.

There are several meditative and relaxation techniques, which are very common. *Yoga-nidrā* is probably a best-known technique to induce the complete physical, mental and emotional relaxation. During the practice of *yoga-nidrā*, the instructor asks the practitioner to visualize certain symbols and images with a witnessing attitude. If the symbols and images are selected properly, then they are in accordance with the symbols of the unconscious. An abstract association is created between the guided imagery and the associated repressed experiences of the unconscious. For example, if the teacher instructs the practitioner to visualize the river or swimming pool, this may bring out a past traumatic childhood experience in which the practitioner was fallen into the river or swimming pool. The practitioner observes this associated painful experience with a witnessing attitude, which helps in cutting off the personal identification with the experience. When the personal identification ceases to cut-off, the painful experience associated with the dog is repressed again. In this way, the practice of visualization brings the unconscious repressed desires, experiences, conflicts and frustrations to the conscious level and then cuts off the personal identification with those experiences. As a result, the unconscious is cleared up.

Due to excessive activity on the mental plane, the mind always remains in a state of arousal, which results in mental tension. Throughout life the mind is fed with negative data. In the practice of *yoga-nidrā*, especially in rotation of consciousness and breath awareness, the mind is relaxed, thereby releasing the mental tensions. In this way, through the regular and sincere practice of *yoga-nidrā*, tensions at the physical, emotional and mental level can be minimized.

"Regression" is a term coined by Galton for the tendency of the quantitative traits of offspring to be closer to the population mean than their parents' traits. It arises from a combination of factors — dominance, gene interactions, and environmental influences on traits.

It is the return to earlier or younger behaviour and thinking. Trauma often overwhelms everyday defences and brings about behavioural regression. Child personality states are an example of trauma-based regression. In "age regression", a person experiences him or herself at a specific earlier age. The person does not always return to the age of a child, however; age regression may take a person back a few years earlier in adult life.

Guilt is that quality which renders criminal and liable to punishment; or it is that disposition to violate the law, which has manifested itself by some act already done. The opposite of innocence, it is remorse caused by feeling responsible for some offence.

Arousal is a physiological and psychological state involving the activation of the reticular activating system in the brain stem, the autonomic nervous system and the endocrine system, leading to increased heart rate and blood pressure, and a condition of alertness and readiness to respond.

It is the stimulation of the brain, causing the subject to go from deep to a lighter level of sleep. This can be easily detected during a sleep study as a change in sleep stage. Arousal can be due to low blood oxygen, high blood carbon dioxide, jerky leg movements, or environmental factors such as loud noises.

Fatigue is a temporary loss of strength and energy resulting from hard physical or mental work; "he was hospitalized for extreme fatigue"; "growing fatigue was apparent from the decline in the execution of their athletic skills"; "weariness overcame her after twelve hours and she fell asleep". It is the point at which the muscle cells are no longer working efficiently. It can be due to depletion of the body's glucose stores, reversible with oral glucose supplements, but also glucose independent, related to changes in the muscle cell itself.

The previous and recent studies show that researchers are very keen to know the physiological and psychological effects of *yoga-nidrā*. It is therefore appropriate now to move from the preliminary exploratory stage to deep into the search through proper controls and predetermined statistical analysis.

Stratified-quota sampling has been used in this study. The total sample covered for the purpose of the present study belonged to the students of PG Yoga classes from Dev Sanskriti Vishwavidyalaya, Shantikunj, Haridwar; who were of 20-30 age group and 110 in numbers (fifty-five males and fifty-five females). They were further divided into forty males and forty females in experimental group; as well as fifteen males and fifteen females in control group.

In the study, control-group research design was adopted. To measure the test psychological parameters — regression, guilt, arousal and fatigue — we have applied the Eight State Questionnaire, developed by Barton, Cattell and Curran in 1973 and adopted by S.D. Kapoor (published and reprinted in India by The Psycho Centre, New Delhi).

Hypothesis and Result

HYPOTHESIS 35

The practice of *yoga-nidrā* will decrease the regression of the male subjects.

Table 15.1: Regression Level of Male Subjects

	Mean	sd	"t" Value	Sig. Level
Experimental	4.95	1.26	2.48	At 0.01
Control	5.67	1.23		

Table 15.1 shows that the post-mean values of the experimental and control groups are 4.95 and 5.67, respectively, and the "t" value is 2.48; there is a significant change at 0.01 significance level in the regression of the male subjects of the experimental and control groups; thus Hypothesis 35 has been proved.

HYPOTHESIS 36

The practice of *yoga-nidrā* will decrease the regression of the female subjects.

Table 15.2: Regression Level of Female Subjects

	Mean	sd	"t" Value	Sig. Level
Experimental	4.62	1.04	2.74	At 0.01
Control	5.80	1.86		

Table 15.2 shows that the post-mean values of the experimental and control groups are 4.62 and 5.80, respectively, and the "t" value is 2.74; there is a significant change at 0.01 significance level in the regression of the female subjects of the experimental and control groups; thus Hypothesis 36 has been proved.

Graph 15.1 shows the post-mean values of regression of the experimental and control groups.

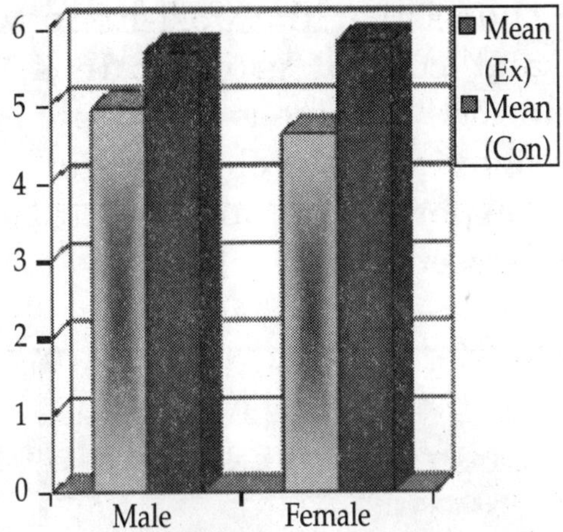

Graph 15.1: Regression

HYPOTHESIS 37

The practice of *yoga-nidrā* will decrease the guilt of the male subjects.

Table 15.3: Guilt Level of Male Subjects

	Mean	sd	"t" Value	Sig. Level
Experimental	4.56	1.12	3.75	At 0.01
Control	5.33	2.13		

Table 15.3 shows that the post-mean values of the experimental and control groups are 4.56 and 5.33, respectively, and the "t" value is 3.75; there is a significant change at 0.01 significance level in the guilt of the male subjects of the experimental and control groups; thus Hypothesis 37 has been proved.

HYPOTHESIS 38

The practice of *yoga-nidrā* will decrease the guilt of the female subjects.

Table 15.4: Guilt Level of Female Subjects

	Mean	sd	"t" Value	Sig. Level
Experimental	4.49	1.50	4.62	At 0.01
Control	5.60	1.35		

Table 15.4 shows that the post-mean values of the experimental and control groups are 4.49 and 5.60, respectively, and the "t" value is 4.62; there is a significant change at 0.01 significance level in the guilt of the female subjects of the experimental and control groups; thus Hypothesis 38 has been proved.

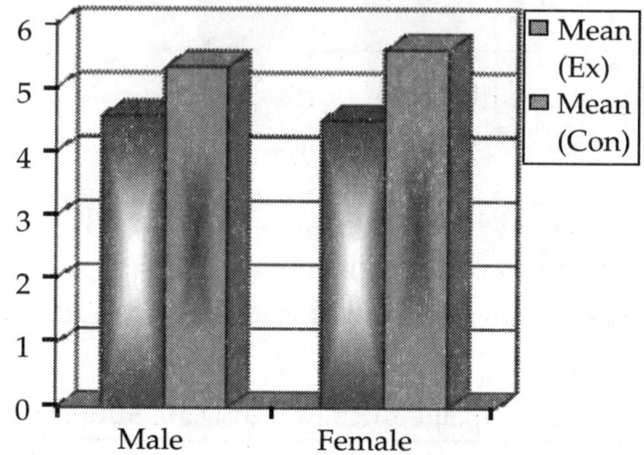

Graph 15.2: Guilt

Graph 15.2 shows the post-mean values of guilt of the experimental and control groups.

HYPOTHESIS 39

The practice of *yoga-nidrā* will decrease the arousal of the male subjects.

Table 15.5: Arousal Level of Male Subjects

	Mean	sd	"t" Value	Sig. Level
Experimental	5.03	1.07	3.2	At 0.01
Control	5.87	1.03		

Table 15.5 shows that the post-mean values of the experimental and control groups are 5.03 and 5.87, respectively, and the "t" value is 3.2; there is a significant change at 0.01 significance level in the arousal of the male subjects of the experimental and control groups; thus Hypothesis 39 has been proved.

HYPOTHESIS 40

The practice of *yoga-nidrā* will decrease the arousal of the female subjects.

Table 15.6: Arousal Level of Female Subjects

	Mean	sd	"t" Value	Sig. Level
Experimental	4.68	1.05	3.8	At 0.01
Control	6.20	0.68		

Table 15.6 shows that the post-mean values of the experimental and control groups are 4.68 and 6.2, respectively, and the "t" value is 3.8; there is a significant change at 0.01 significance level in the arousal of the female subjects of the experimental and control groups; thus Hypothesis 40 has been proved.

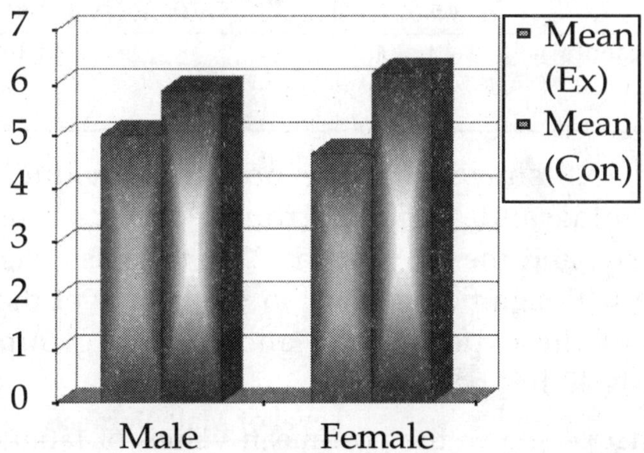

Graph 15.3: Arousal

Graph 15.3 shows the post-mean values of arousal of the experimental and control groups.

HYPOTHESIS 41

The practice of *yoga-nidrā* will decrease the fatigue of the male subjects.

Table 15.7: Fatigue Level of Male Subjects

	Mean	sd	"t" Value	Sig. Level
Experimental	4.70	0.94	1.12	At 0.01
Control	4.80	1.01		

Table 15.7 shows that the post-mean values of the experimental and control groups are 4.7 and 4.8, respectively, and the "t" value is 1.12; there is a significant change at 0.01 significance level in the fatigue of the male subjects of the experimental and control groups; thus Hypothesis 41 has been proved.

HYPOTHESIS 42

The practice of *yoga-nidrā* will decrease the fatigue of the female subjects.

Table 15.8: Fatigue Level of Female Subjects

	Mean	sd	"t" Value	Sig. Level
Experimental	4.43	0.96	2.17	At 0.01
Control	4.80	0.77		

Table 15.8 shows that the post-mean values of the experimental and control groups are 4.43 and 4.8, respectively, and the "t" value is 2.17; there is a significant change at 0.01 significance level in the fatigue of the female subjects of the experimental and control groups; thus Hypothesis 42 has been proved.

Graph 15.4 shows the post-mean values of fatigue of the experimental and control groups.

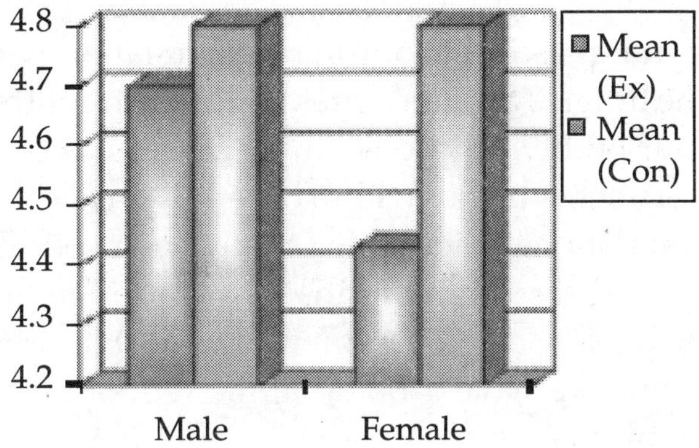

Graph 15.4: Fatigue

Conclusion

A significant change also has been observed in the regression, guilt, arousal and fatigue of the subjects during this study. When the individual fails to adjust to the situation, distress results. Some individuals are prone to developing distress due to their unconscious urge to remain tense. When distress continues for a long period, it may result in psychological disorders like neuroses or even psychoses. In the practice of *yoga-nidrā*, the inherent tendency to become tense is rooted out and the individual starts viewing the situation as less demanding. Gersten (1978) said that the practitioner of *yoga-nidrā* becomes his own psychotherapist, recognizing and systematically alleviating his own personal problems and interpersonal difficulties. Matthew (1981) reported that *yoga-nidrā* is a successful therapy for both recent and long-standing psychological disturbances of all kinds, especially high anxiety levels and neurotic behaviour patterns. Shealy (1998) concluded that *yoga-nidrā* is a successful treatment for insomnia. In this manner, various researches show that the technique of *yoga-nidrā* can be successfully administered to manage various psychological disorders. As the previous studies show that practice of *yoga-nidrā*, meditation and relaxation significantly lowers all the psychological problems, it supports the findings of the present study.

There is no question about the close relation between the body and the brain. Various centres in the brain control, modify and affect our bodily functions. In fact, there is a centre in the brain for every act, whether willful or reflex, physical or mental. Experimental data have identified many such specific centres. Stimulation of these centres leads to appropriate actions, be they motor or sensory, secretary or emotive, affective or cognitive. Thus we have a holographic representation of the body on the brain.

To put the thing more concretely, it is proved that the left half of the body is represented by the right half of the brain and vice versa. As far as the muscular actions are concerned, the representation is in an "upside–down manner" in motor area of pre-central *gurus*. Thus, at the top of this part of brain the lowest portion of our body — foot — is represented. Then comes ankle, leg (calf), knee, thigh, hip, trunk, shoulder, arm, elbow, wrist, palm, fingers, thumb, then neck, jaw, face, eyes, ears, tongue, etc. The same thing is applicable for sensations. Stimulation of brain centres of sensory cortex evokes sensations on the opposite half of the body.

In *yoga-nidrā* exactly opposite process is used to make the brain centres active by focusing awareness on the parts of the body in a definite sequence. Thus, the person tries to stimulate various parts of the brain by focusing the awareness on the corresponding parts of the body. By awareness is meant the "attitude of witness" towards physical or mental actions of the body.

16

Effect of Yoga-Nidrā on Hypertension

HYPERTENSION is an important and a common risk factor for considerable morbidity and mortality not only in the industrialized world but also in the developing countries. Thus, the problem of hypertension can be truly considered as pandemic. It is an increased pressure of blood results from the damming up of blood behind constricted arterioles, upsetting the balance of the heart and its vessels.

Hypertension is described by Maharṣi Suśruta as *śira-kuñcan* and *rakta-pūrṇatā.*

कुर्यात्सिरागतः शूलं सिराऽऽकुञ्चनपूरणम्।
kuryāt sirāgataḥ śūlaṁ śirā ''kuñcan pūraṇam

> The wind/air contained in the blood vessels produces pain and constriction of arterioles and venules due to provocation and thus raises tension of blood form within.
>
> – *Suśruta Saṁhitā,* Nidāna sthāna 1.27

In the modern world, mind-related diseases like hypertension, stress and schizophrenia are quite common. Tension is the central theme of all mind-related diseases. This tension is due to the strain of life that an individual carries. It is well established that the brain with its known centres for sensory, intellectual and emotional tensions play the main role in maintaining by liberating required amount of neurohumors and hormones. Any disorder of this homeostatic by any factor would ultimately lead to the development of tension. Related therapies have been unable to answer the question of prevention and cure of hypertension.

Now comes the practice of *yoga* to combat this most prevalent disease. Although there are many relaxation and meditation techniques available to the common people, something was lacking to deal with hypertension properly. *Yoga-nidrā* is probably the best-known technique to induce complete physical, mental and emotional relaxation. *Yoga-nidrā* is a state of consciousness, which is, neither sleep nor awaken, neither is it concentration nor hypnotism. It can be defined, as an altered state of consciousness.

Yoga-nidrā is a state of magnetism. In the state of *yoga-nidrā* the whole body is magnetized and it becomes full of electromagnetic pulsation, vibration and concentration. With these phenomena, the body becomes painless, respiration becomes occasional, and the heart rate slows down, according to the stimulation or depression of the cardiac centre in the medulla oblongata.

Carrington et al. (1980) have concluded in their work that *yoga-nidrā* has its widespread application as a preventive measure, to be practised by healthy active people as a means of relieving accumulated tensions, increasing stress resistance and overall of psychosomatic disease.

Another controlled study, done by Lekh Raj Bali (1997) which was conducted at the Langley Porter Neuropsychiatry Institute in California, found that there is a reduction in blood pressure and anxiety levels in hypertensive patients continues for twelve months after the *yoga-nidrā* training.

An American pilot, with a six-year old history of high blood pressure, underwent various treatments without results. Following a six-week programme of *yoga* and relaxation, his blood pressure was normalized and he regained full-flight status. And as the researchers pointed out, relaxation also has an advantage over medicine in that it had no side effects, something which can be hazardous for a fighter pilot.

Material and Methods

Forty patients, suffering from essential hypertension (male = 30, female = 10) of an age group of 30-60 years from same occupation, have been selected for the study through quota-sampling technique. All the males were businessmen and the females were housewives. The study was based on pre- and post-group designing as there was no control group and the directional hypothesis has been applied. The study has been conducted at Pataliputra Seva Sansthan, Patna City, Patna. Duration of the study was fifteen days and the practice time was 30 minutes.

Yoga-nidrā practised in this study is the easiest method of relaxation. It is being practised in the flat-lying position of *śavāsana* and follows the spoken instruction of the *yoga*-instructor. It is convenient to use *yoga-nidrā* tape. The practice includes the stages — preparation, resolve, body part awareness, breath awareness visualization and ending of the practice.

Tools applied for the study were sphygmomanometer for blood pressure measurement, stopwatch — for pulse rate and respiration rate — and a general questionnaire developed with the help of the guide of this project work, Swami Mangalteertham Saraswati, Prof. and Head, Applied Yogic Science, Bihar Yoga Bharti, Munger, for other psychological correlates.

Hypothesis and Result

HYPOTHESIS 43

The practice of *yoga-nidrā* will positively decrease the systolic blood pressure of the subjects.

Table 16.1: Systolic Blood Pressure Level of the Subjects

	Mean	sd	"t" Value
Pre	155	15.38	10.13
Post	125	10.28	

Table 16.1 shows the means of the pre- and post-values as 155 and 125, respectively, and the "t" value as 10.13 at 0.01 significance levels. Thus Hypothesis 43 has been proved.

HYPOTHESIS 44

The practice of *yoga-nidrā* will positively decrease the diastolic blood pressure of the subjects.

Table 16.2: Diastolic Blood Pressure Level of the Subjects

	Mean	sd	"t" Value
Pre	98	11.16	8.09
Post	76	12.78	

Table 16.2 shows the means of the pre- and post-values as 98 and 76, respectively, and the "t" value as 8.09 at 0.01 significance levels. Thus Hypothesis 44 has been proved.

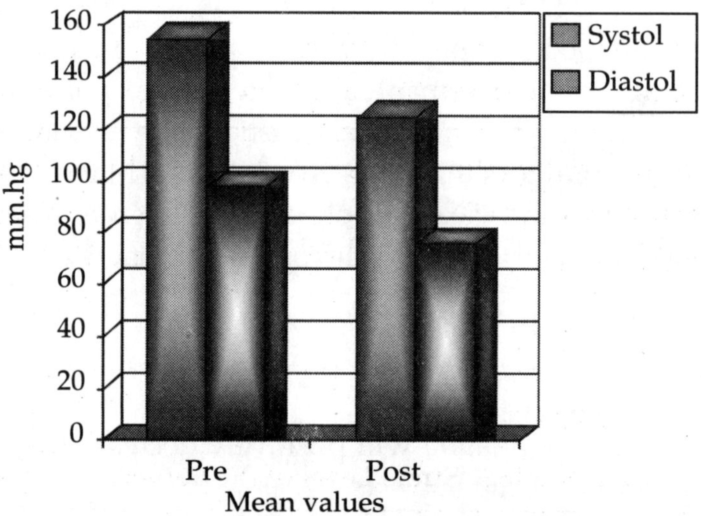

Graph 16.1: Blood Pressure

Graph 16.1 shows the pre- and post-values of systolic and diastolic blood pressure of the subjects having mild hypertension, practised *yoga-nidrā*.

HYPOTHESIS 45

The practice of *yoga-nidrā* will positively decrease the pulse rate of the subjects.

Table 16.3: Pulse Rate of the Subjects

	Mean	sd	"t" Value
Pre	84	7.87	6.47
Post	73	7.13	

Table 16.3 shows the means of the pre- and post-values as 84 and 73, respectively, and the "t" value as 6.47 at 0.01 significance level. Thus Hypothesis 45 has been proved.

HYPOTHESIS 46

The practice of *yoga-nidrā* will positively decrease the respiratory rate of the subjects.

Table 16.4: Respiration Rate of the Subjects

	Mean	sd	"t" Value
Pre	27.5	5.25	5.02
Post	22.13	4.10	

Table 16.4 shows the means of the pre- and post-values as 27.5 and 22.13, respectively, and the "t" value as 5.02 at 0.01 significance level. Thus Hypothesis 46 has been proved.

HYPOTHESIS 47

The practice of *yoga-nidrā* will positively decrease the stress level of the subjects.

Table 16.5: Stress Level of the Subjects

	Mean	sd	"t" Value
Pre	2.3	0.87	8.12
Post	1.0	0.14	

Table 16.5 shows the means of the pre- and post-values as 2.3 and 1, respectively, and the "t" value as 8.12 at 0.01 significance level. Thus Hypothesis 47 has been proved.

HYPOTHESIS 48

The practice of *yoga-nidrā* will positively decrease the fear level of the subjects.

Table 16.6: Fear Level of the Subjects

	Mean	sd	"t" Value
Pre	1.50	1.09	3.57
Post	0.75	0.17	

Table 16.6 shows the means of the pre- and post-values as 1.5 and 0.75, respectively, and the "t" value as 3.57 at 0.01 significance level. Thus Hypothesis 48 has been proved.

HYPOTHESIS 49

The practice of *yoga-nidrā* will positively decrease the anger level of the subjects.

Table 16.7: Anger Level of the Subjects

	Mean	sd	"t" Value
Pre	2.15	1.07	4.76
Post	1.05	0.80	

Table 16.7 shows the means of the pre- and post-values as 2.15 and 1.05, respectively, and the "t" value as 4.76 at 0.01 significance level. Thus Hypothesis 49 has been proved.

HYPOTHESIS 50

The practice of *yoga-nidrā* will positively decrease the depression level of the subjects.

Table 16.8: Depression Level of the Subjects

	Mean	sd	"t" Value
Pre	2.0	0.88	0.96
Post	0.9	0.66	

Table 16.8 shows the means of the pre- and post-values as 2 and 0.9, respectively, and the "t" value as 0.96 at 0.01 significance level. Thus Hypothesis 50 has been rejected.

Conclusion

Hypertension is not a disease *per se*, but a syndrome of multiple diseases. In most of the cases the causes remain silent.

However, *yoga-nidrā* can be considered as a highly effective practice for reducing blood pressure of hypertensive patients on the basis of the present study. It has been found that *yoga-nidrā* reduces the pulse rate, respiration rate and also releases the stress, fear and anger of the hypertensive people. Through the body–mind relationship, relaxation of body relaxes the entire nervous system. Through the relaxation of central nervous system in *yoga-nidrā* relaxation in autonomic nervous system takes place, and it reduces the whole physical and mental activities. Reduction in the muscular and neural activities slows down the metabolic rate of the body.

During the practice of *yoga-nidrā,* due to the relaxed body and mind, muscles become relaxed and the arteries become dilated as vasodilation occurs. Hence the cardiac output as well as cardiac workload reduce; the systolic and diastolic blood pressure with pulse rate, comes down as has been seen in the present study.

Due to the practice of *yoga-nidrā* relaxed body requires less oxygen, accordingly less metabolic activities. Need of the oxygen in the body becomes less; due to that, reduction in the respiration rate has been observed. *Yoga-nidrā* didn't show a significant change in the depression level of the patients, and thus we know that the practice of *yoga-nidrā* is not beneficial for a depressed person. As the previous studies also support our study, the practice of *yoga-nidrā* can be considered as an effective tool to be introduced as a preventive measure to control hypertension.

17

Suggestions for Further Researches

THOUGH the utmost care was taken in formulating the design and of conduction the study, it cannot be said with confidence that the study was perfect in all aspects. Therefore, it is the humble duty of the investigator to point out the limitations of the study so that further investigations could improve in the right direction.

Options are available everywhere. All these studies of the effect of *yoga-nidrā* are on few psychological and few physiological parameters. Here we have included almost all common psychological and few hematological parameters.

In future, some more different psychological and physiological parameters can be taken for a new study. The previous works were long-term studies as they were based on six months duration. One of the studies is very short as it is based on fifteen days observation only. In future, a short-term study can be conducted which should not be less than forty days.

It covers only a specific age group as the subjects are of 20-30 age group. In future, the new study may involve a different age group. This study involves only the physically fit persons as subject; in future persons suffering from different disorders can be taken as subjects.

The present investigation was done to study the effect of the *yoga-nidrā* on human physiology and psychology. The techniques applied in drawing the samples were from one institution; better results could be obtained by applying this technique in various institutions.

These studies were based on the specific technique of *yoga-nidrā* which is based on the teachings of Swami Satyananda

Saraswati. During the study we modified the instruction as per the need of the situation. As the study conducted on higher-class students; the visualization part of the practice had to be changed for a good result of the study so that the creativity and concentration could be increased as well as examination stress and phobias could be released. It is being suggested that the practice of *yoga-nidrā* should be varying from person to person. In future it is being suggested that the researcher, without changing the basic instructions of the practice of *yoga-nidrā*, can change the visualization part of the *yoga-nidrā*.

In these studies dependent variables were more. It is suggested that for better results less variables can be taken in further researches. It is further suggested on the basis of this study that if one has to work on any specific psychological or physiological parameter, the visualization should be changed as per the demand of the study.

18

Experience the Yoga-Nidrā

YOGA-NIDRĀ means psychic sleep. Sleep rests the body, but *yoga-nidrā* rests both the mind and body. When you are asleep, your consciousness sleeps in your astral body, but in *yoga-nidrā* your consciousness is awake within. *Yoga-nidrā* performs two beneficial functions. It removes fatigue and invigorates the body. The stresses and strains of daily life create tensions and these rob the mind of its serenity. *Yoga-nidrā* removes tensions and restores the elasticity of your mind.

The evils of day-to-day life are deposited in our subconscious mind and in due course they exert a deleterious influence on our mental make-up. Just as our house must be swept daily to keep it tidy, to have a normal personality, we must remove the *saṁskāra*s, the mental dirt that accumulates daily in our subconscious mind. *Yoga-nidrā* performs this essential service for us, removing our mental abnormalities and clearing the way to spiritual progress.

How to practise *yoga-nidrā*? First do a few *āsana*s and *prāṇāyāma*s and follow them up with *yoga-nidrā*. This technique is best learned from a *guru*. Not that it will harm you if you practise it without his help, but if you do it on your own, the chances are that every time you begin you will end up falling asleep. Then the *saṁskāra*s will not be destroyed and you will not make any progress. To be absolutely successful, *yoga-nidrā* presupposes a spirit of communion between the *guru* and the disciple. Only that disciple who has complete reverence for the *guru* can obtain the benefits of *yoga-nidrā*.

Yoga-nidrā should not be practised immediately after meals. Mentally sick persons should practise it three times a day for longer durations, say for one hour each session, after a preparatory round of *āsanas* and *prāṇāyāmas*. *Trāṭaka* will increase the efficacy if practised before *yoga-nidrā*, but if it is found to be too difficult, then *śāmbhavī-mudrā* or *nāsikāgra dṛṣṭi* can be done. If these preliminaries are performed, the *guru* is in a better position to help the disciple. *Yoga-nidrā* is a psycho-physiological therapy.

What is *yoga-nidrā*? It is a state in which you are neither asleep nor awake. If you fall asleep, it is not *yoga-nidrā*. If you remain awake, then too it is not *yoga-nidrā*. If dreams overtake you, it is not *yoga-nidrā*. *Yoga-nidrā* is a state in which there is awareness of the conscious, subconscious and unconscious fields of your mind all at one time. It is a perfect therapy. It removes all psychological abnormalities and *saṁskāras*, and helps you to become your normal, natural self.

Patañjali has defined *yoga* as the control of the *citta-vṛttis* (mental modifications). Good behaviour is the outcome of the *citta-vṛttis*; similarly, bad behaviour is also the outcome of the *citta-vṛttis*. Our conscious, subconscious and unconscious fields are our *citta*. Simultaneous awareness of these three fields is *aham asmi* or (I am). This state in which you are aware but not aware that you are aware comes in *yoga-nidrā*. Thereafter a process of sure but imperceptible sublimation takes place within.

It is said that meditation creates a fire which burns away our sins. What is sin? Actions which create uneasiness and abnormal feelings in the mind are sins. Cynics dismiss the word sin with a smile of derision. Whenever your conscience pricks you for any of your actions, that action is sin. Cynics are no exception to this rule; sin is there whether they admit it or not. In meditation your consciousness penetrates the various layers of your inner self. This is the fire that burns away the dross of *saṁskāras* within. Thereafter comes the yogic state of supreme peace and tranquillity of mind described in the second chapter of the *Bhagavad-Gītā*.

Yoga-nidrā is one of the main techniques for the attainment of this peace. The most important point in *yoga-nidrā* as well as in other meditation practices is that you must not allow yourself to fall asleep. In *yoga-nidrā,* sleep tries to overpower you. If you can overcome this weakness, you will gain in willpower, and through will-power you can do great things in your life. If sleep comes, concentrate on the body or on the sleep itself as if it is trying to possess you and you are watching it. If images arise before your mind, go on watching them. In

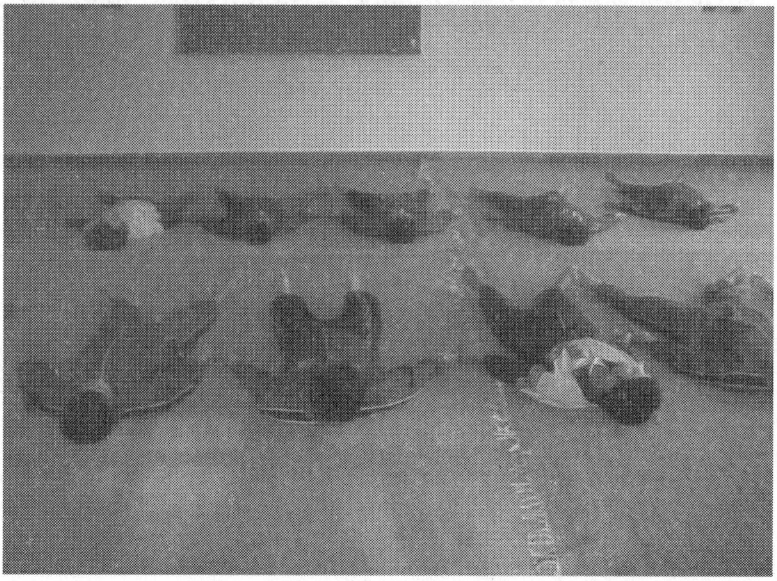

fig. 18.1: Yoga-Nidrā (practice)

yoga-nidrā, when you feel that you are unconscious, it actually means that you are conscious of being unconscious.

Those who follow the *guru*'s instructions implicitly in *yoga-nidrā* are assured of success. Circumstances or worldly ties are not hindrances to spiritual progress. The only hindrances are your own ignorance and sloth. We must make the blessings of *yoga-nidrā* as widely known as possible. Many mental and physical disorders of both young and old are cured by *yoga-nidrā*. It is a psychosomatic technique and could do immense good to our children if educational institutions were to include it in their curriculum.

To experience the *yoga-nidrā* one should follow the instruction mentioned below.

Preparation

Lie down in *śavāsana* with legs apart and hands beside the body while palm facing upward. Head, neck and spine should be in one line. Close your eyes and relax the body. During the practice of *yoga-nidrā* you don't have to fall in sleep and don't have to move the body. Just feel that you are in complete rest for sleep but don't sleep. Observe the body parts, observe the bodily condition and observe the outer environment. Observe the sounds coming from outside the room.

Saṅkalpa

The practice includes resolution (*saṅkalpa*). Take a positive resolution related to the goal of life. Repeat it three times mentally. Resolution should be short and simple.

Rotation of Consciousness

Now start rotating the awareness in body parts. Start with right side of the body right hand thumb, index finger, middle finger, ring finger, little finger, palm, back of the palm, right wrist, forearm, elbow, upper arm, shoulder, armpit, right side chest, waist, right hip, right thigh, knee, ankle, right big toe, second toe, third toe, forth toe, fifth toe and the whole right side. Bring the awareness to the left side of the body — left hand thumb, index finger, middle finger, ring finger, little finger, palm, back of the palm, left wrist, forearm, elbow, upper arm, shoulder, armpit, left side chest, waist, left side hip, left thigh, knee, ankle, left big toe, second toe, third toe, forth toe, fifth toe and the whole left side of the body. Bring the awareness now to the back part of the body — both the soles, heels, calf muscles, back of the knees, back of the thighs, both the buttocks, hip joint, lower back, upper back, spine, shoulder blades, back of the neck, back of the head. Bring the awareness to the front part of the body. Top of the head, forehead, eyebrows, eyes, ears, nostrils, cheeks, lips, chin, throat, chest, upper abdomen, lower abdomen, hip joint, thighs, knee cap, shin bone, feet and the whole front part of the body. Now observe the whole body at once.

Breath Awareness

Bring the awareness now to your breath, no change in breathing pattern. Just watch the natural breath. Observe the movement at the abdominal region, the navel comes up and goes down. Just count down the breath starting from twenty-three and reach up to zero. No hurry, no mistake. If you forget the number, again start with twenty-three. Be aware that you are practising *yoga-nidrā,* don't fall asleep. Be aware of the breath, be aware of the number.

Visualization

Leave the awareness of breath, start visualize the thing as per instruction — just feel that the body weight is increasing and you are becoming heavy, pause, just feel that the body weight is losing and you are becoming light weighted, pause, feel the coolness of the environment, pause, feel the hotness of the environment. Try to visualize the rising sun, pause, the candle flame, pause, the full moon, pause, the stars in the sky, pause. . . . heavy raining . . . red clouds . . . the flying birds . . . endless desert . . . deep well . . . small garden . . . sea burning fire. . . . *Oṁ* . . . statue of Lord Buddha. . . . Mahākāla. . . . etc.

Saṅkalpa

Let the visualization end; repeat the resolution three times again. Repeat the same *saṅkalpa* with full faith.

Ending

Start moving the toes and fingers, hands, legs and neck. Move the body slowly, turn to the left and come up into seated position with eyes closed. Rub the palm and keep it on the eyes. Open eyes slowly. *Yoga-nidrā* ends.

Yoga-nidrā is a superlative relaxation tool but, the true purpose of *yoga-nidrā* goes well beyond deep relaxation. *Yoga-nidrā* establishes the link between the conscious desires, the will-power, the subconscious and the unconscious mind. When this happens one reaps all-round powerful benefits and feels the total control on all aspects of life.

Bibliography

Agras, W.S. (1980), "Relaxation Training: Twenty-four Hour Blood Pressure Reduction", *Arch. Gen. Psychiat.*, 37: 859-63.

Agrawal, R.S. (2009), "Yoga Nidra: An Open Secret of Divine Yogic Self Healing Technique", *Chartered Accountant*, 58(5): 847.

Amita, S. et al. (2009), "Effect of Yoga Nidra on Blood Glucose Level in Diabetic Patients", *Indian Journal of Physiol. & Pharmacol*, **53** (1), 97-101.

Bahrke, M.S. (1979), "Exercise, Meditation and Anxiety Reduction: A Review", *Amer. Corr. Ther. J.*, 32(2): 41-44.

Bali, Lekh Raj (1979), "Long-term Effect of Relaxation on Blood Pressure and Anxiety Levels of Essential Hypertensive Males: A Controlled Study", *Psychosom. Med.*, 41(8): 119-204.

Baron, Robert A. (2000), *Psychology*, 3rd edn., New Delhi: Prentice Hall of India.

Bevan, James (1994), *A Pictorial Handbook of Anatomy & Physiology*, London: Reed International Books.

Bhushan, S. (2006a), "Qualitative Transformation in Personality: A Function of Yoga Nidra", *Journal of Indian Psychology*, 24(1/2): 65-75.

——— (2006b), "Yoga-Nidra as Intervenor to Promote Self-Confidence Among Teenagers", *Indian Journal of Psychometry and Education*, 37(1): 11-16.

——— (2007), "Qualitative Transformation in Personality: A Function of Yoga Nidra", *Journal of Indian Psychology*, 25(1/2): 6-15.

Bhushan, Siddhartha and Pammi Sinha (2001), "Yoga-Nidra and Management of Anxiety and Hostility", *Journal of Indian Psychology*, 19: 44-49.

Brownstein, A.H. and M. L. Dembert (1998), "Treatment of Essential Hypertension with Yoga Relaxation Therapy in a USAF Aviator: A Case", *Bindu*, no. 11 Haa Course Center, 34013 Hamneda, Sweden.

Carrington, P. et al. (1980), "The Use of Meditation-Relaxation Techniques for the Management of Stress in a Working Population", *J. Occup. Med.*, 22(4): 221-31.

Cooper, M.J. and M.M. Aygen (1979), "A Relaxation Technique in the Management of Hypercholesterolemia", *J. Hum. Stress*, 5(a), pp. 24-27.

Datey, K.K. and S.J. Bhagat (1977), "Stress and Heart Disease and How to Control It with Biofeedback and Shavasana", *Quart. J. Surg. Sci.* (Banaras Hindu University), 13: 3-4.

Deuskar, M., N. Poonawala, S.A. Bhatewara (2006), "Effect of Yoga Nidra and Applied Relaxation Technique on Steadiness and Performance of Archers", *Psychological Studies*, 51(1): 64-68, University of Calicut.

Erskine-Milliss, J. and M. Schonell (1981), "Relaxation Therapy in Asthma: A Critical Review", *Psychosom. Med.*, 43(4): 365-72.

Evelin C. Pearce (1993), *Anatomy & Physiology for Nurses*, 16th edn., New Delhi: Jaypee Brothers.

Flak, M. (1978), "Teaching Yoga to Children", *Yoga*, 16(2), Munger: Bihar School of Yoga.

Gersten, D.J. (1978), "Meditation as an Adjunct to Medical and Psychiatric Treatment", *Amer. J. Psychiat.*, 135: 5.

Goel, Arun (2001), *Understanding Deep Relaxation Through Yoga Nidra*; www.healthandYoga.com.

Gupta, G.B., G.C. Sepaha, I. Menou and S.K. Tiwari (1979), "The Effects of Yoga on Bronchial Asthma", *Yoga*, 27(2): 29-33.

Gupta, L.P. et al. (2000), *Positive Health Though Ayurveda*, Chaukhambha Sanskrit Prakashan.

Jansson, L. (1979), "Behavioral Treatment of Irritable Colon", *Scand. J. Behav. Ther.*, 8(4): 119-204.

Macey, Jennifer (2005), "Stress in relation to immunity", *Journal of Experimental Medicine*, 202(11): 1456-82.

Khushbu Rani et al. (2012), "Yoga-Nidra as a Complementary Treatment of Anxiety and Depressive Symptoms in Patients with Menstrual Disorder", 5(1): 52-56.

Kumar, Kamakhya (2004), "Yoga-Nidra and Its Impact on Student's Well-being", *Yoga Mīmāṁsā*, 36(1): 31-35, Lonavla: Kaivalyadhama.

——— (2005), "Effect of Yoga-Nidra on Hypertension and Other

Psychological Co-relates", *Yoga the Science*, 3(7), Hubli (Karnataka): Yoga Publications, pp. 70-78.

——— (2006), "A Study on the Improvement of Physical and Mental Health Through Yoga Nidra", *Dev Sanskriti Journal* (4): 39-46.

——— (2007), "The Healing Sleep", *Yoga Magazine Mind Body Spirit*, London-York Street, Issue 50, March, pp. 42-44.

——— (2008), "A Study on the Impact on Stress and Anxiety through Yoga-Nidra", *Indian Journal of Traditional Knowledge*, 7(3): 401-04.

——— (2010), "Psychological Changes as Related to Yoga-Nidra", *International Journal of Psychology: A Biopsychosocial Approach*, 6: 129-37.

Kumar, Kamakhya and Bhanu Joshi (2009), "Study on the Effect of Pranakarshan Pranayama and Yoga-Nidra on Alpha EEG and GSR", *Indian Journal of Traditional Knowledge*, 8(3): 453-54.

Kumar Kamakhya and Pranav Pandya (2012), "A Study on the Impact on ESR Level Through Yogic Relaxation Technique Yoga Nidra", *Indian Journal of Traditional Knowledge*, 11(2): 358-61.

Mandlik, Vishwas, Yogacharya, Premchand Jain, Kiran M.S. Jain (2002), *Effect of Yoga Nidra on EEG (Electro-Encephalo-Graph)*, Nasik, Maharastra: Yoga Vidyadham.

Mangalteertham, Sannyasi (A.K. Gosh) (1998), "Yoga Nidra: Altered State of Consciousness", *Yoga Nidra*, Munger: Bihar School of Yoga, 6th edn., pp. 245-53.

Matthew, R.J. (1981), "Anxiety and Platelet MAO Levels After Relaxation Training", *Amer. J. Psychiat.*, 138(3): 371-73.

Meares, A. (1979), "Regression of Cancer of the Rectum after Intensive Meditation", *Med. J. Aust.*, 2(10): 539.

Meares, A. (1980), "Remission of Massive Metastases from Undifferentiated Carcinoma of the Lung Associated with Intensive Meditation", *J. Amer. Soc. Psychosom, Dent. & Med.*, 27(2): 40-41.

Medicalcenter.osu.edu/patientcare/healthinformation/otherhealthtopics/ArthritisOtherRheumaticDi4155/ArthritisandOtherRheumati4181.

Nespor, K. (1981), "Prevention of Cardiovascular Diseases from a Psychosomatic Point of View", *Cas. Lek. Ces.*, 120(35): 1055-58, repr. in *Yoga* (Bihar School of Yoga).

Nilsson, Robert (1997-98), "Pictures of the Brain's Activity During Yoga Nidra", *Bindu*, no. 11, Haa Course Center, 34013 Hamneda, Sweden.

Ostrander, S. and L. Schroeder (1973), *Psi: Psychic Discoveries Behind the Iron Curtain*, Abacus, UK, pp. 290-302.

Panda N.C. (2007), *Yoga-Nidra Yogic Trance: Theory, Practice and Applications* (first published in 2003), New Delhi: D.K. Printworld, pp. 191-92.

Pandya, Pranav, *Akhand Jyoti*, November-December 2003; p. 37, November-December 2004, pp. 7, 10.

Pandya, Pranav and Kamakhya Kumar (2007), "Yoga-Nidra and its Impact on Human Physiology", *Yoga Vijñāna*, **1**(1): 1-8.

Pritchard, M., P. Elison-Bowers, B. Birdsall (2010), "Impact of Integrative Restoration (iRest) Meditation on Perceived Stress Levels in Multiple Sclerosis and Cancer Outpatients", *Stress and Health*, **26**(3): 233-37.

Rama (Swami) (1988) *Path of Fire and Light*, vol. II, USA: Himalayan Institute Pub.

Rani, K. et al. (2011), "Impact of Yoga-Nidra on Psychological General Wellbeing in Patients with Menstrual Irregularities: A Randomized Controlled Trial", *Int. J. Yoga* [serial online] [cited 19 April 2011], 4: 20-25.

Rasal, S. and M. Deuskar (2008), "Effectiveness of Rational Emotive Therapy (RET) and Yoga Nidra for Anger Management in Families", *Psychological Studies*, **53** (3/4): 213-18.

Roney-Dougal, S.M. (2001), *Altered States of Consciousness and Yogic Attainment in Relation to Awareness of Precognitive and Clairvoyant Targets*; Psi Research Center.

Saraswati, (Swami) Muktibodhanda (1985, 2000), *Hath Yoga Pradipika*, Munger: Bihar School of Yoga, p. 467.

Saraswati, (Swami) Niranjananada (1995), *Yoga Darshan*, Munger: Bihar School of Yoga, p. 115.

——— (1993, 2001), *Yoga Darshan*, Munger (Bihar): Yoga Publication Trust.

Saraswati, (Swami) Satyananda (1975, 1998, 2001); *Dynamics of Yoga*, Munger: Yoga Publication Trust.

——— (2001), *Yoga Nidra*, Munger: Yoga Publication Trust.

Sealy R.C. (1979), *The Effectiveness of Various Treatment Techniques on*

Different Degrees and Durations of Sleep-onset Insomnia, Behav Res Ther, 17:541.

Selye, H. (1974), *Stress Without Distress*, New York: J.B. Lippincott Co.

Sharma, Sriram (Acharya) (1995), *Sādhanā Paddhatiyoṅ kā Gyān aur Vigyān*, Mathura: Akhand Jyoti Sansthan, p. 31.

——— (2001), *Sleep Dream and Spiritual Reflections*, Haridwar: Sri Vedmata Gayatri Trust, Shantikunj.

Shealy, R.C. (1998), "The Effectiveness of Various Treatment Techniques in Different Degrees and Durations of Sleep-onset Insomnia", in Swami Satyananda's *Yoga Nidra*, Munger: Bihar School of Yoga, 6th edn.

Simonton, O.C. (1972), The Role of the Mind in Cancer Therapy. Transcript from the Dimensions of Healing: A Symposium, Academy of Parapsychology and Medicine, Stanford University.

Udupa, K.N. (1977), "Pathogenesis and Management of Stress Disorders," *Quart. J. Surg. Sci.*, 13(2): 56, Banaras Hindu University.

——— (1978, 2000), *Stress and Its Management Through Yoga*, Delhi: Motilal Banarsidas, p. 110.

Verma, Veena (Sannyasi Saumya Shakti) (2004), "Possibilities of Revolutionizing the Education System Through Yoga Nidra", *Yoga* Magzine; published from Bihar School of Yoga, May 2004.

Index